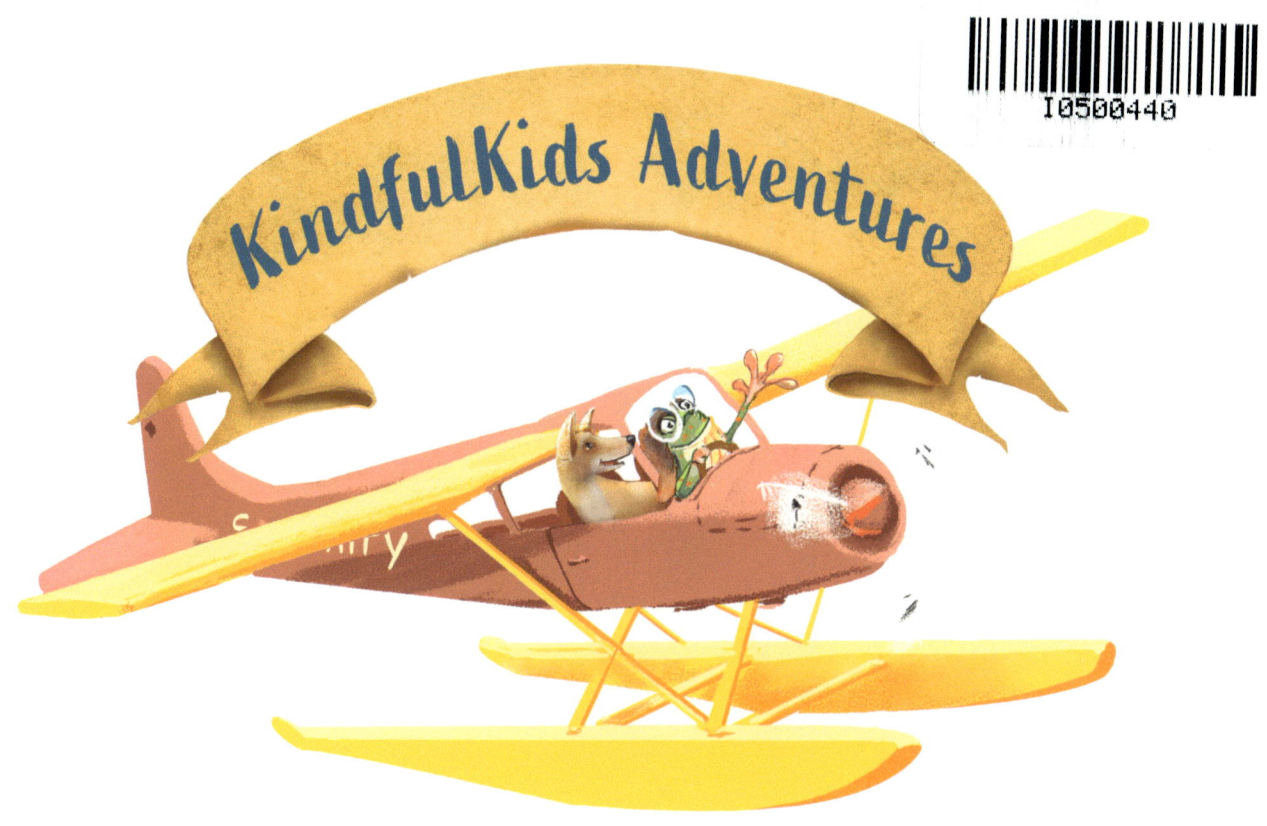

KindfulKids Adventures

Search for Serenity

Written by Patricia Leitch

Illustrated by Soledad Cook

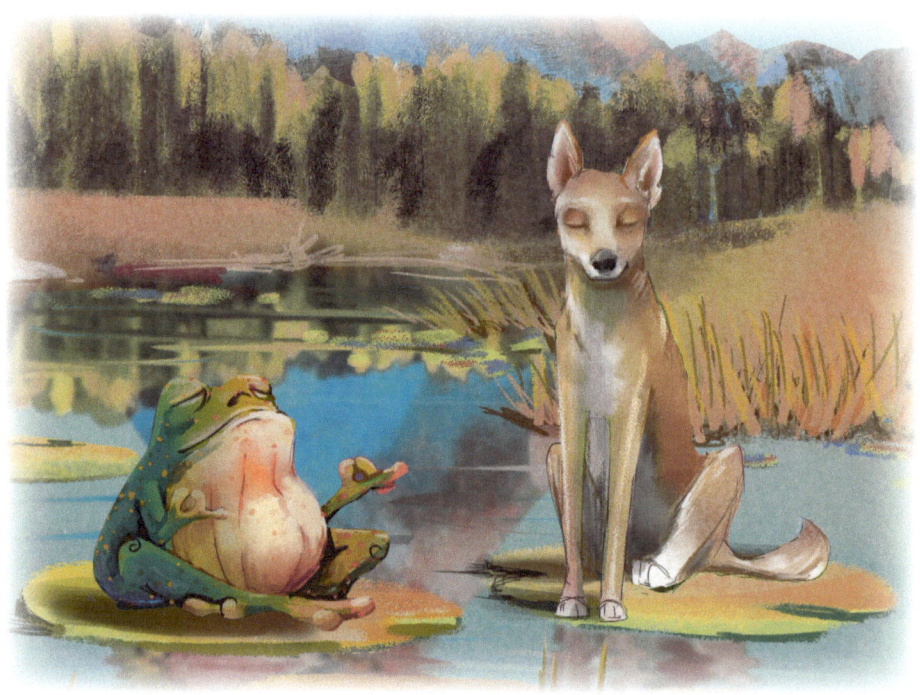

To all the students at Hoover Elementary school.
Thank you for the inspiration.

Search for Serenity
Copyright® 2019
All rights reserved.
Published by Level Above ™ Publishing in the United States of America.
For information, go to kindfulkids.com

ISBN: 978-0-9980349-3-5

Second Edition

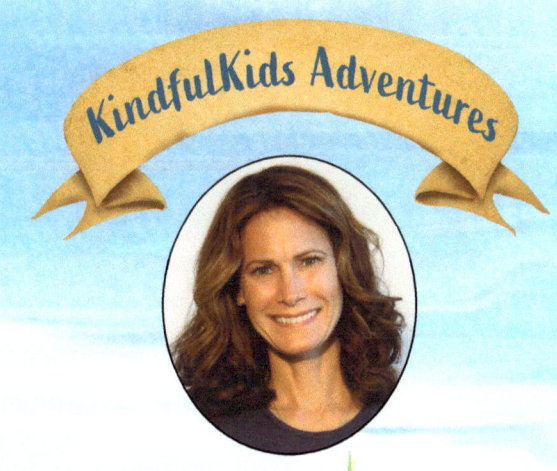

Welcome to *KindfulKids Adventures,*

You have probably heard, introducing mindfulness and meditation to children can impart health benefits that last a lifetime.

BUT, as mother and teacher, I know that encouraging kids to be still and breathe deep is not easy or interesting for them.

I created the KindfulKids series to provide parents and teachers with a fun and engaging way to introduce young children to mindful disciplines.

This book, SEARCH FOR SERENITY, sets kids up to experience the mind body connection that is meditation. The yoga poses help develop breath awareness and the frog leaps increase heart rate. Together they allow children to naturally connect to their breath and body in a positive kinetic way. Synching the mind and breath together is the first step to authentic meditation.

Thank you for creating a generation of KindfulKids.

XO, Patricia

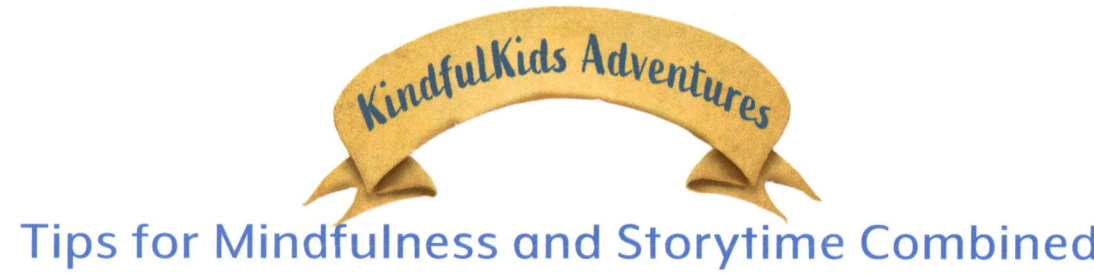

Tips for Mindfulness and Storytime Combined

KindfulKids is about a fun and relaxing experience, not perfect yoga poses. To better accommodate your child's needs, we recommend giving any of the following a try.

◆ Choose a location where you can be face-to-face with your child(ren) with enough space for stretching.

◆ Adapt the story to suit the age and interest of your child:

  · For children under the age of 4, leave out the yoga instructions and simply allow them to find their version of the pose.

  · For children ages 6 and 7, adjust the instructions to their level and interest in holding the yoga poses.

  · For children 8 and up, suggest they instruct younger siblings or friends with the book as a guide.

◆ The most important part of the poses are full deep breaths. If any of the poses are too challenging, skip them or decrease instructional detail.

Learn more about your child's kindful nature by reviewing the questions at the end.

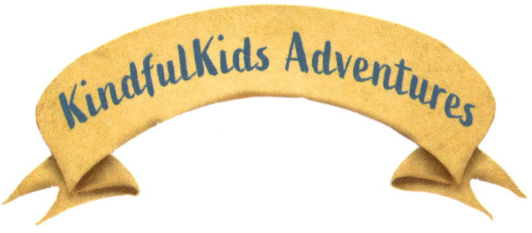

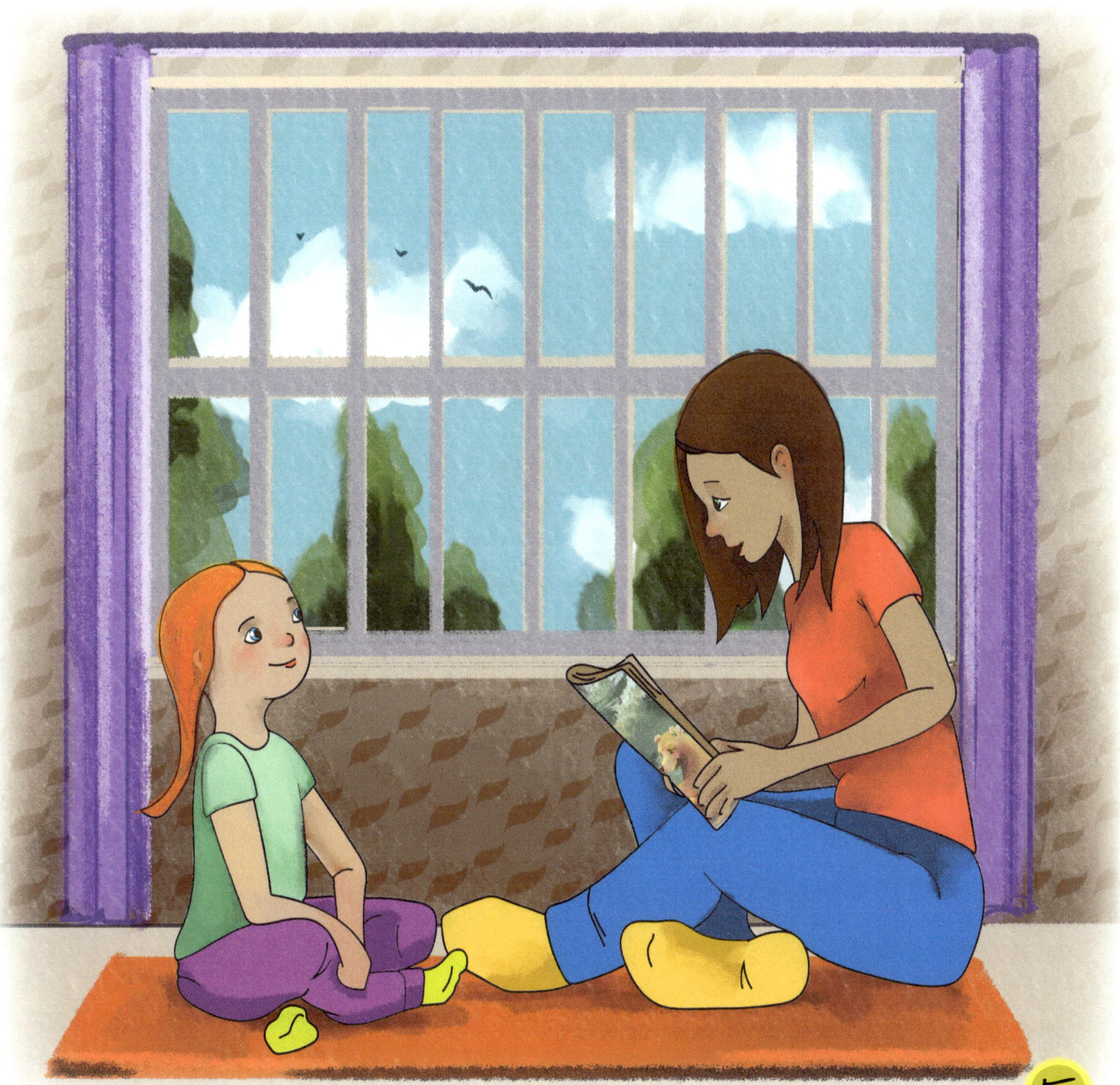

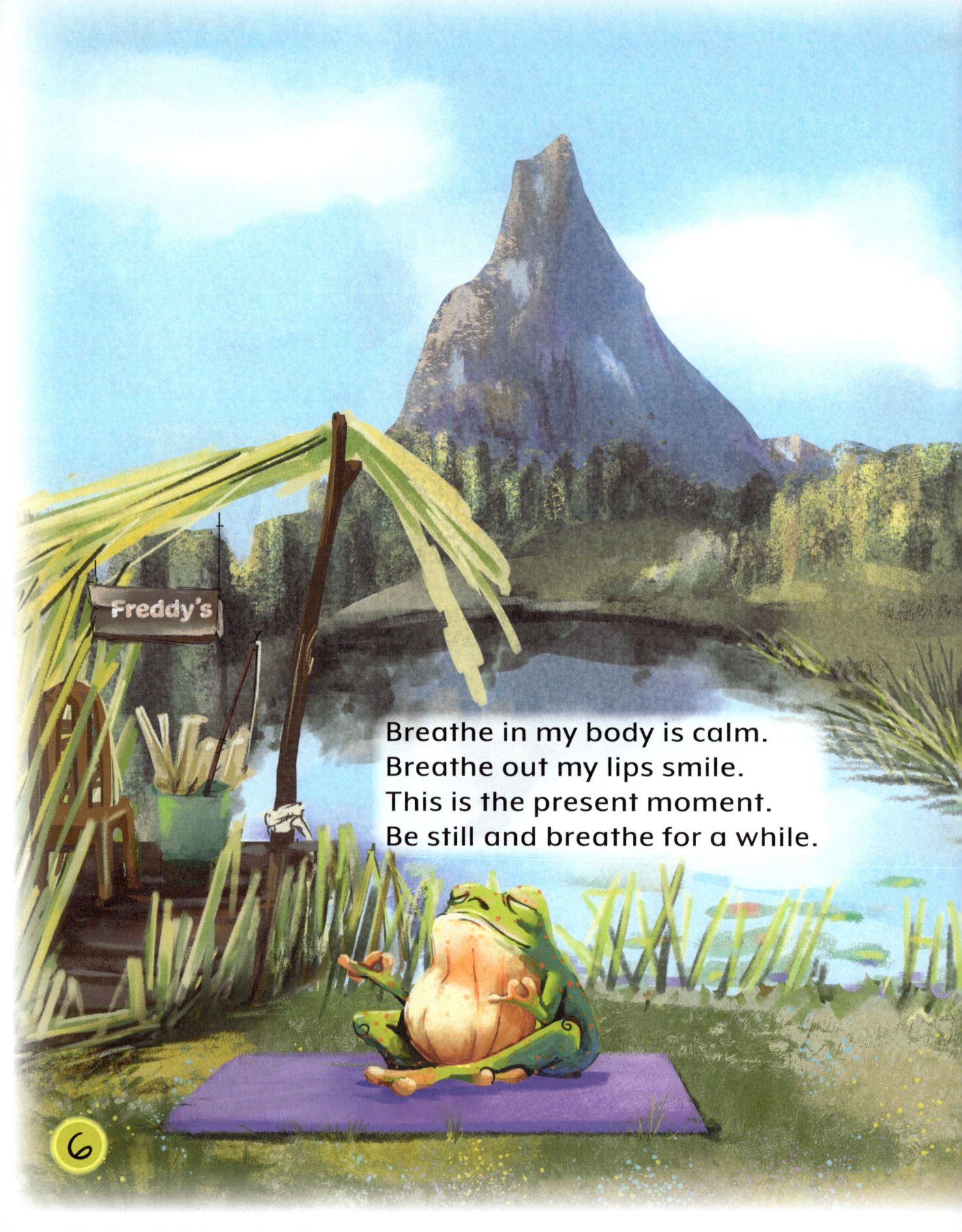

Breathe in my body is calm.
Breathe out my lips smile.
This is the present moment.
Be still and breathe for a while.

Hi kids. It's Danny the Dingo Dog. I am at Pondering Pond and am so excited. My awesome friend Freddy the Frog is taking me for a ride on his seaplane. While I wait for Freddy, will you pratice yoga with me? Cool! Let's start with Sun Salutation.

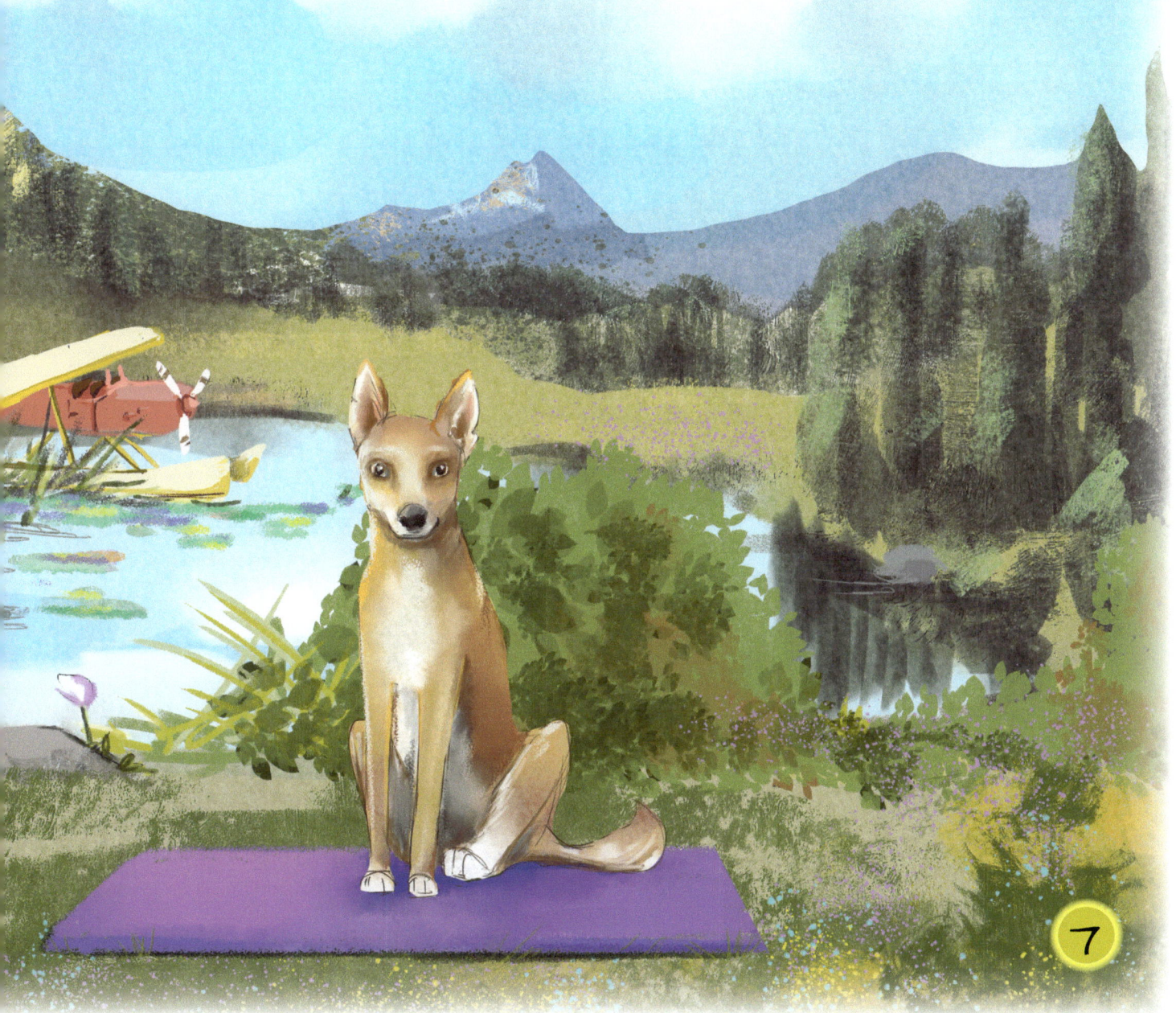

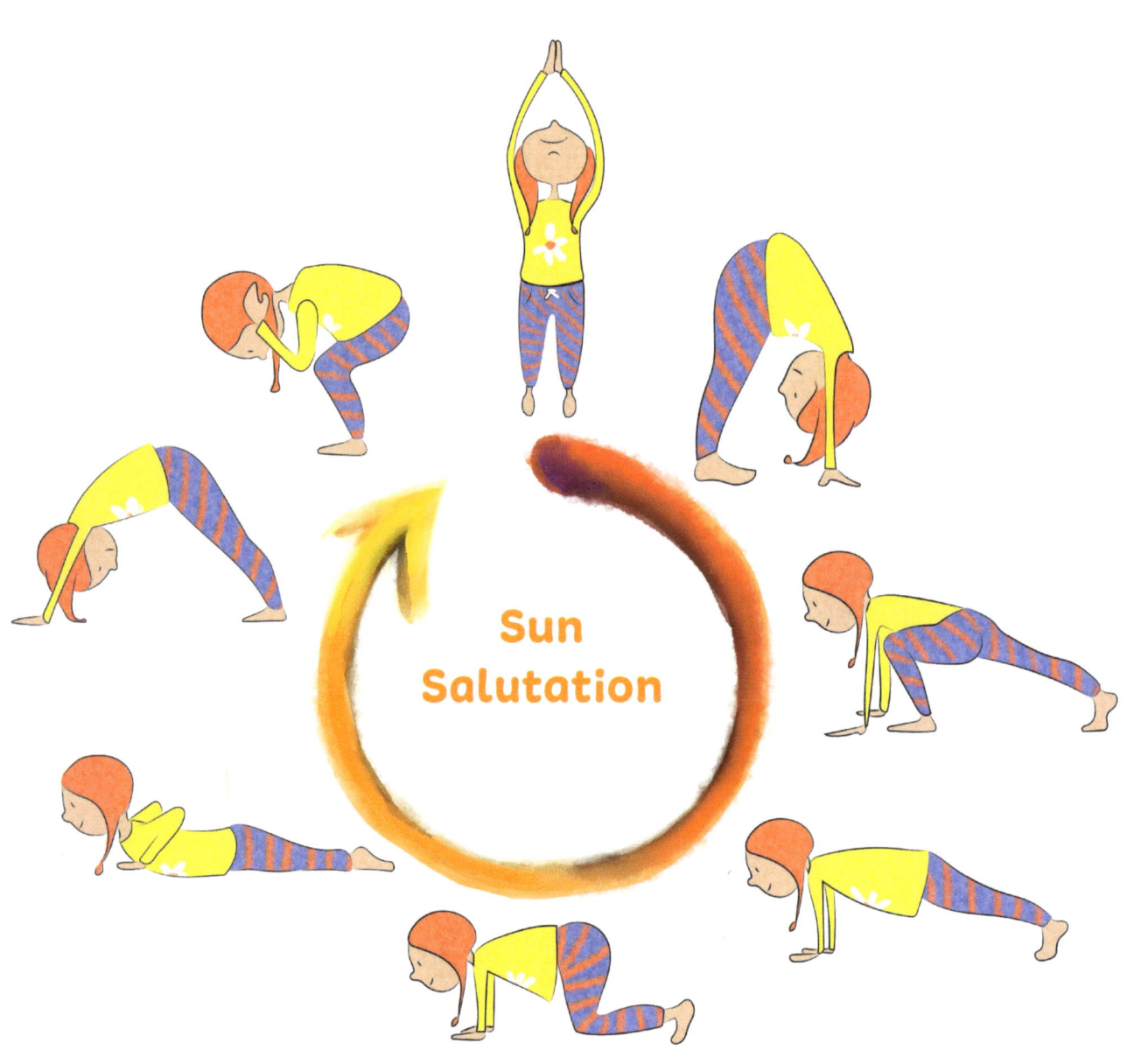

Sun
Salutation

8

Sun Salutation

Inhale, look at hands above your head.

Exhale, place hands in front of your feet.

Inhale, bring one foot then the other back to plank pose.

Exhale, bring your knees then chest to the floor.

Inhale, move your chest forward lift your palms off the ground.

Exhale back to downward facing dog.

Take a few breaths in downward facing dog.

Inhale deeply, exhale fully.

Inhale deeply, exhale fully.

Tippy toe your feet to your hands.

Place your elbows on your knees.

Roll up to return to standing position.

If you like, try Sun Salutation again.

"Freddy," said Danny loudly. "When are we flying? You are just sitting with your eyes closed? What are you doing?"

"It is called meditation," says Freddy. "It's practicing being still. Do you want to try?"

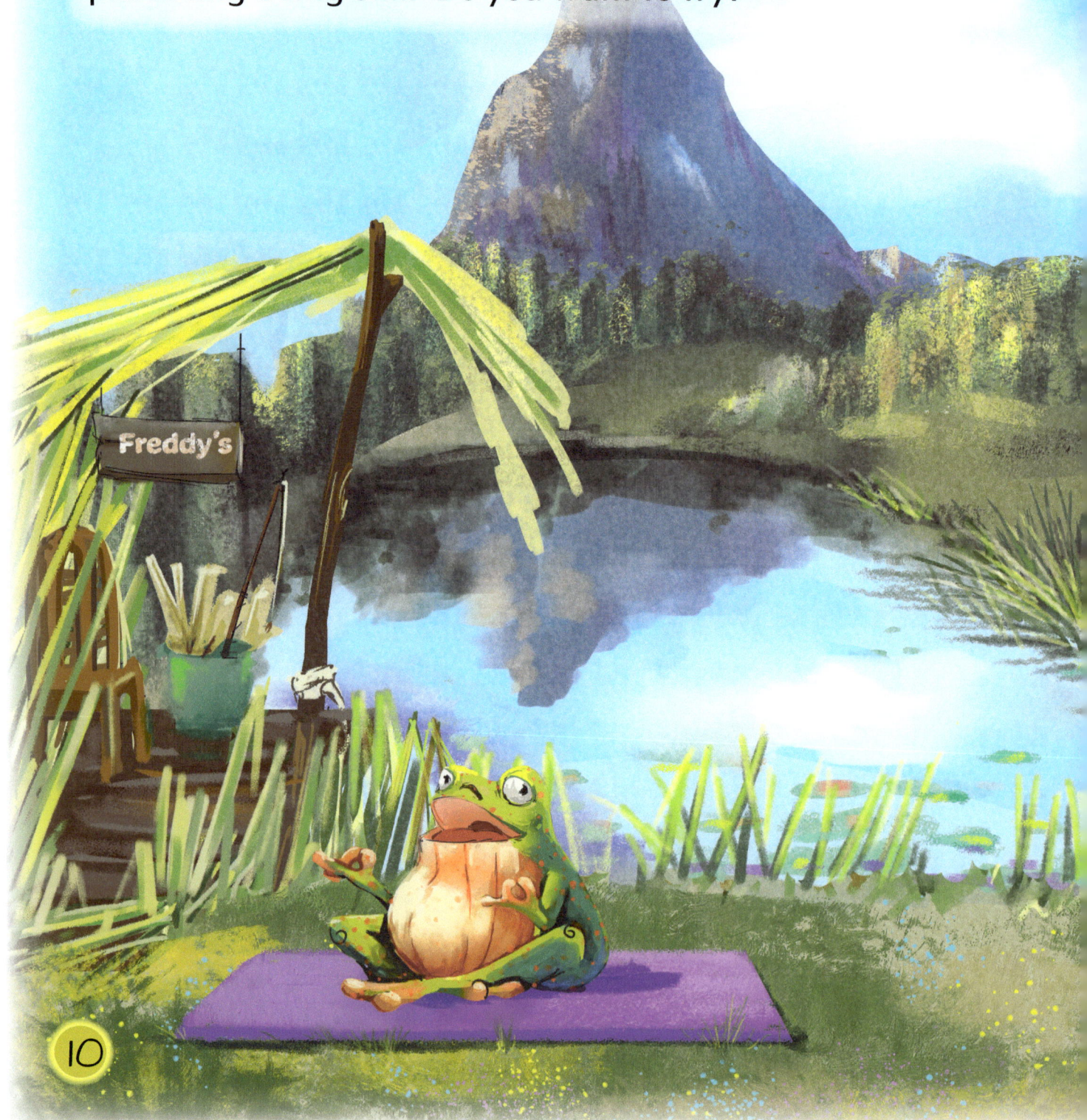

"Meditation? I can't be still and meditate Freddy. I make too many mistakes." Danny replied.

"Alright Danny, then continue your yoga. We will fly soon enough." says Freddy.

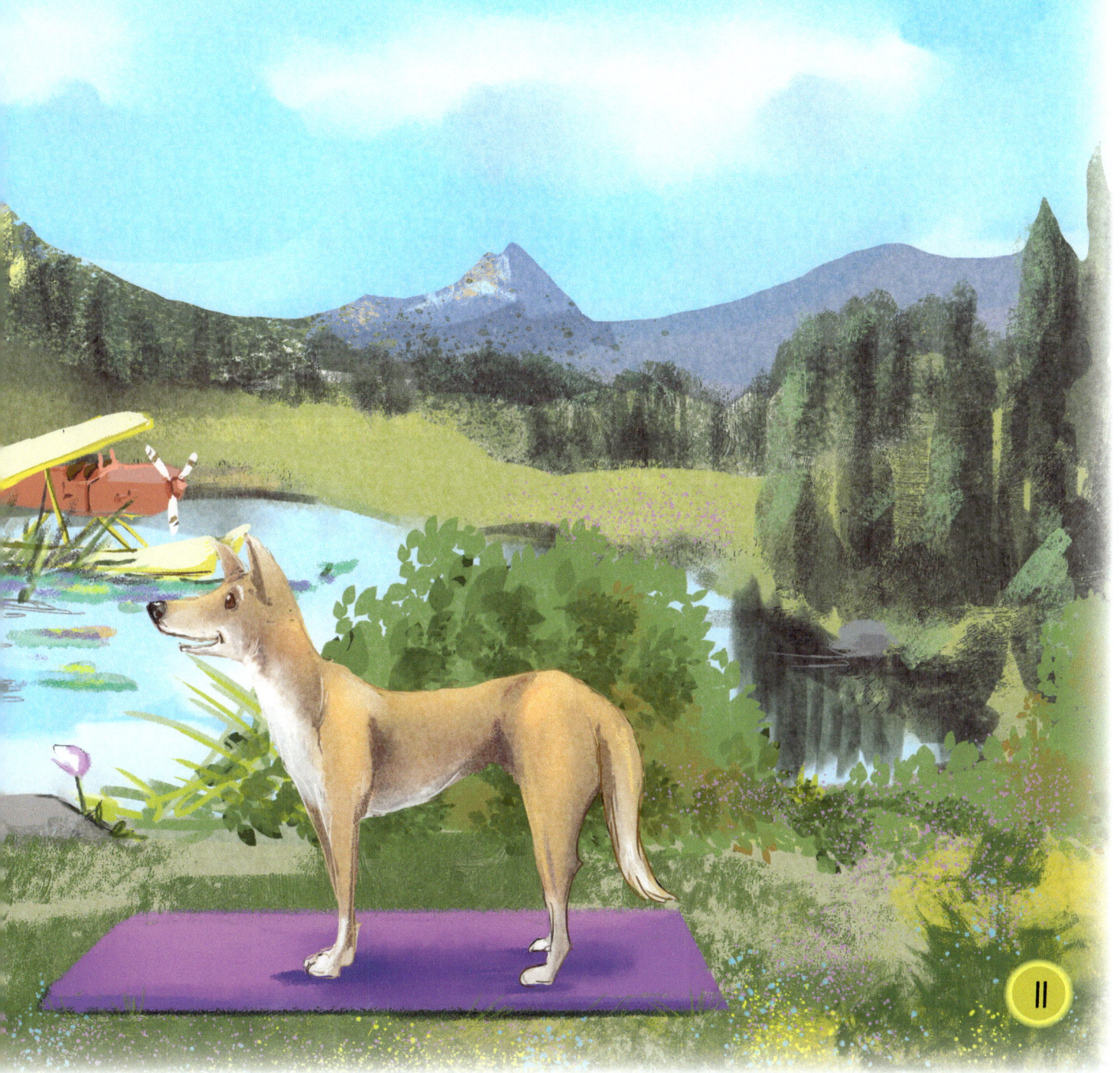

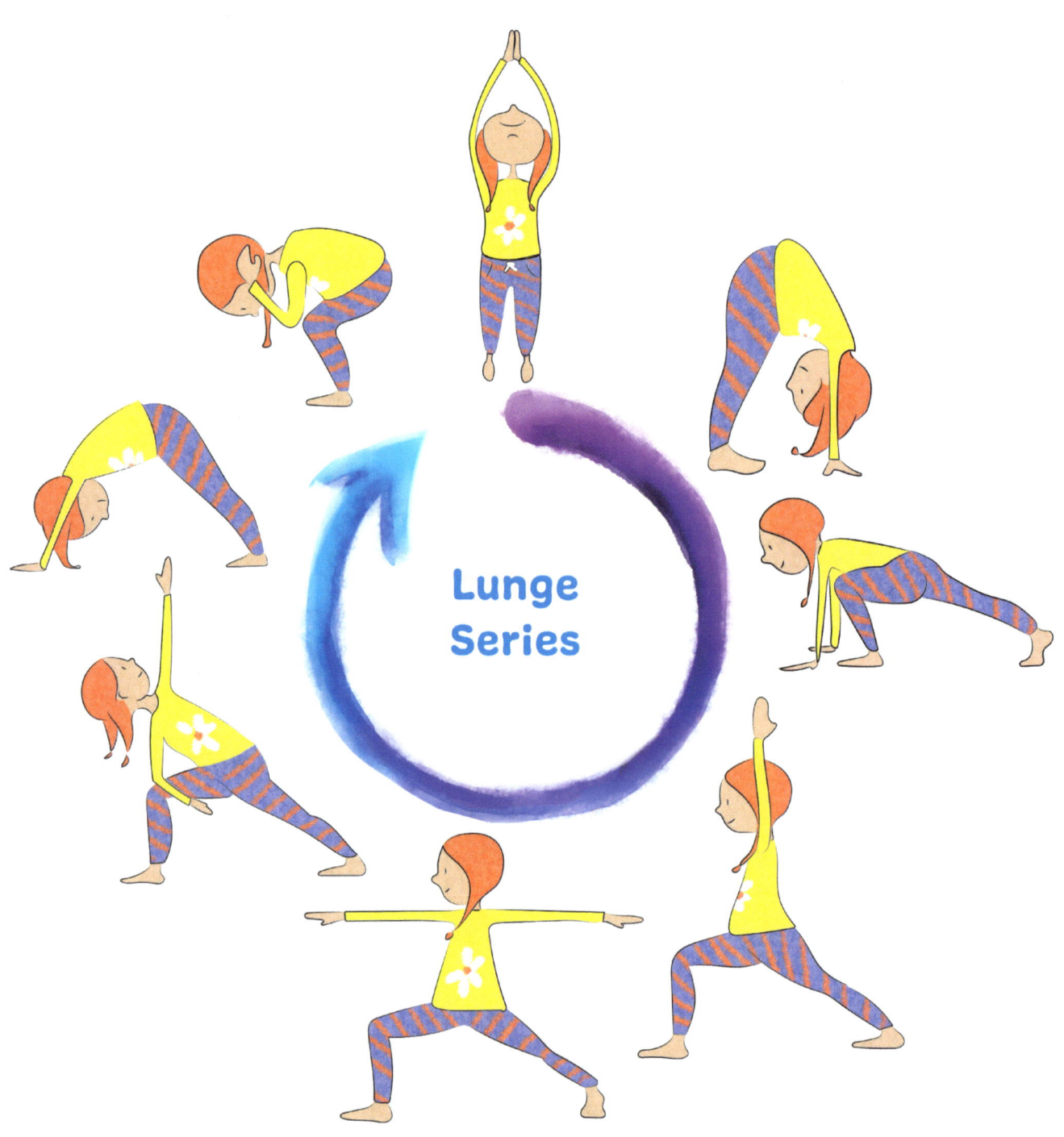

Lunge
Series

Lunge Series

Inhale, bring hands together above your head.

Exhale, bend forward and place hands in front of your feet.

Inhale, bring one leg back with front knee bent.

Exhale, look at your hands on the ground.

Inhale, lift hands above your head into lunge pose.

Exhale, open your arms to the side.

Inhale, bend your front arm at the elbow.

Exhale, place your elbow on your knee and look up at your thumb.

Take a few deep breaths here.

Then return to downward facing dog.

Tippy toe your feet to your hands.

Place your elbows on your knees.

Roll up to return to standing position.

Try this lunge series on the other leg.

"Freddy, wouldn't flying be more fun than yoga or meditation?" says Danny.

"Well, it is a beautiful day, and I've finished my practice." Let's get into my seaplane and go for a ride."

"So excited! Finally I get to fly in the sky," says Danny.

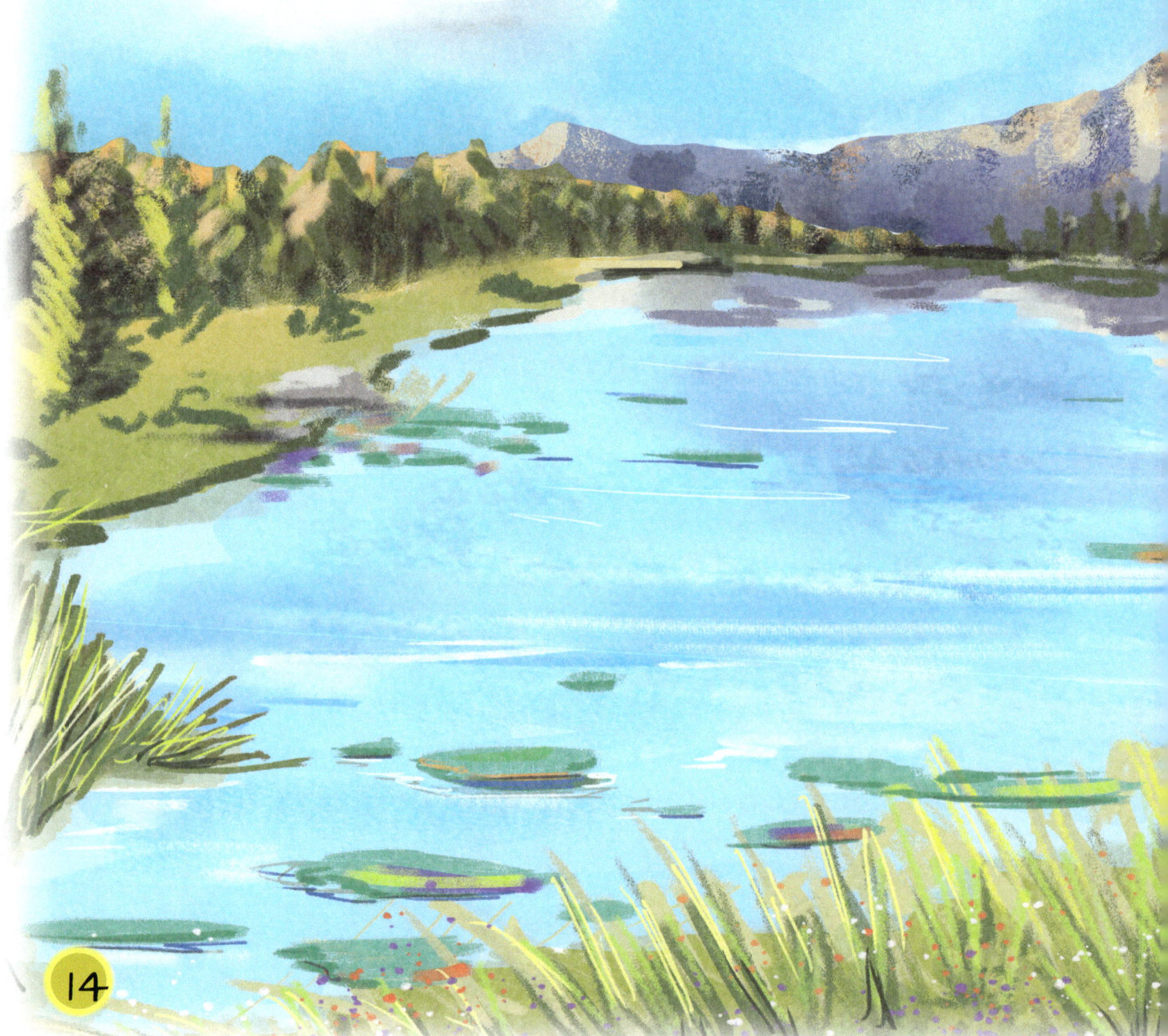

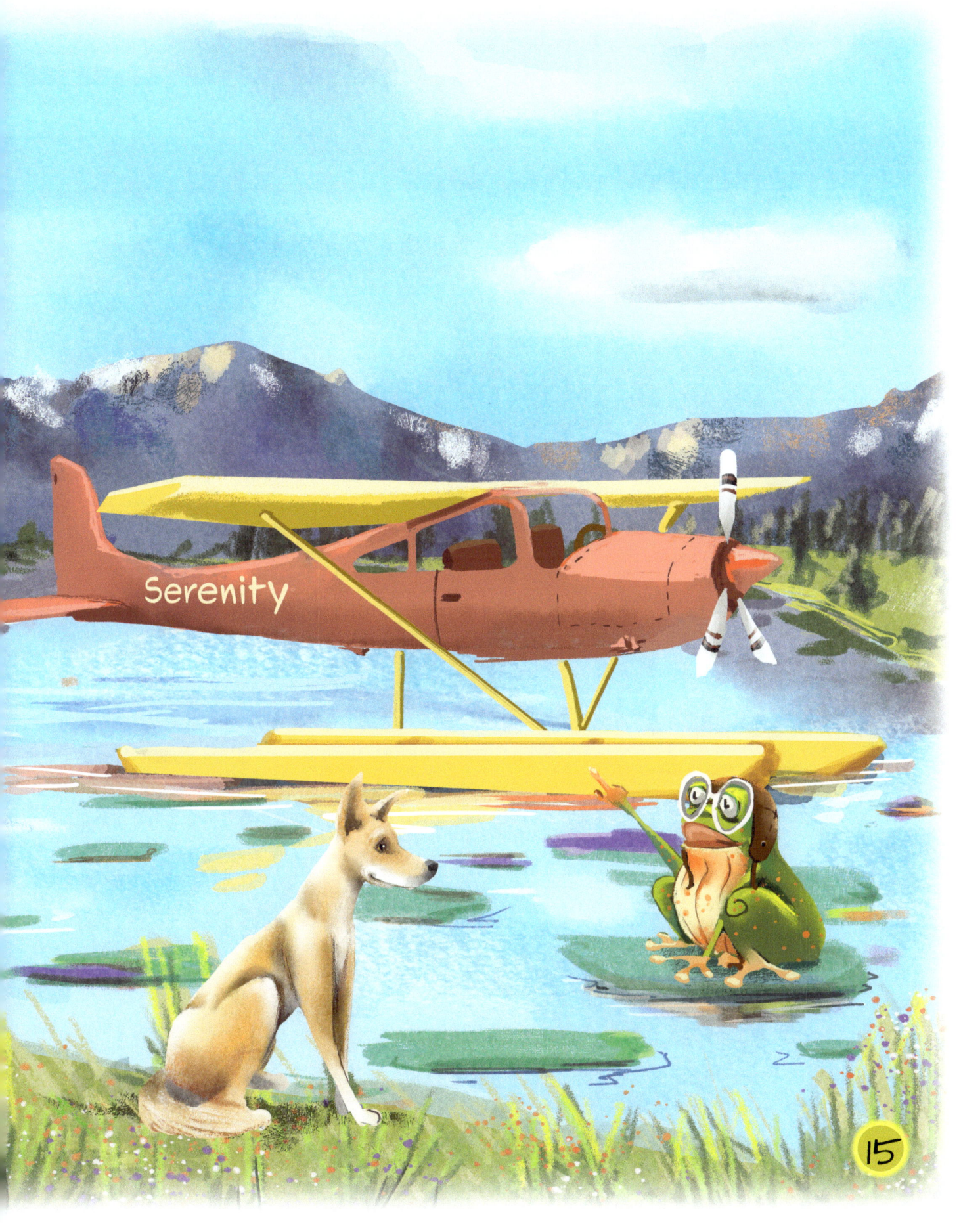

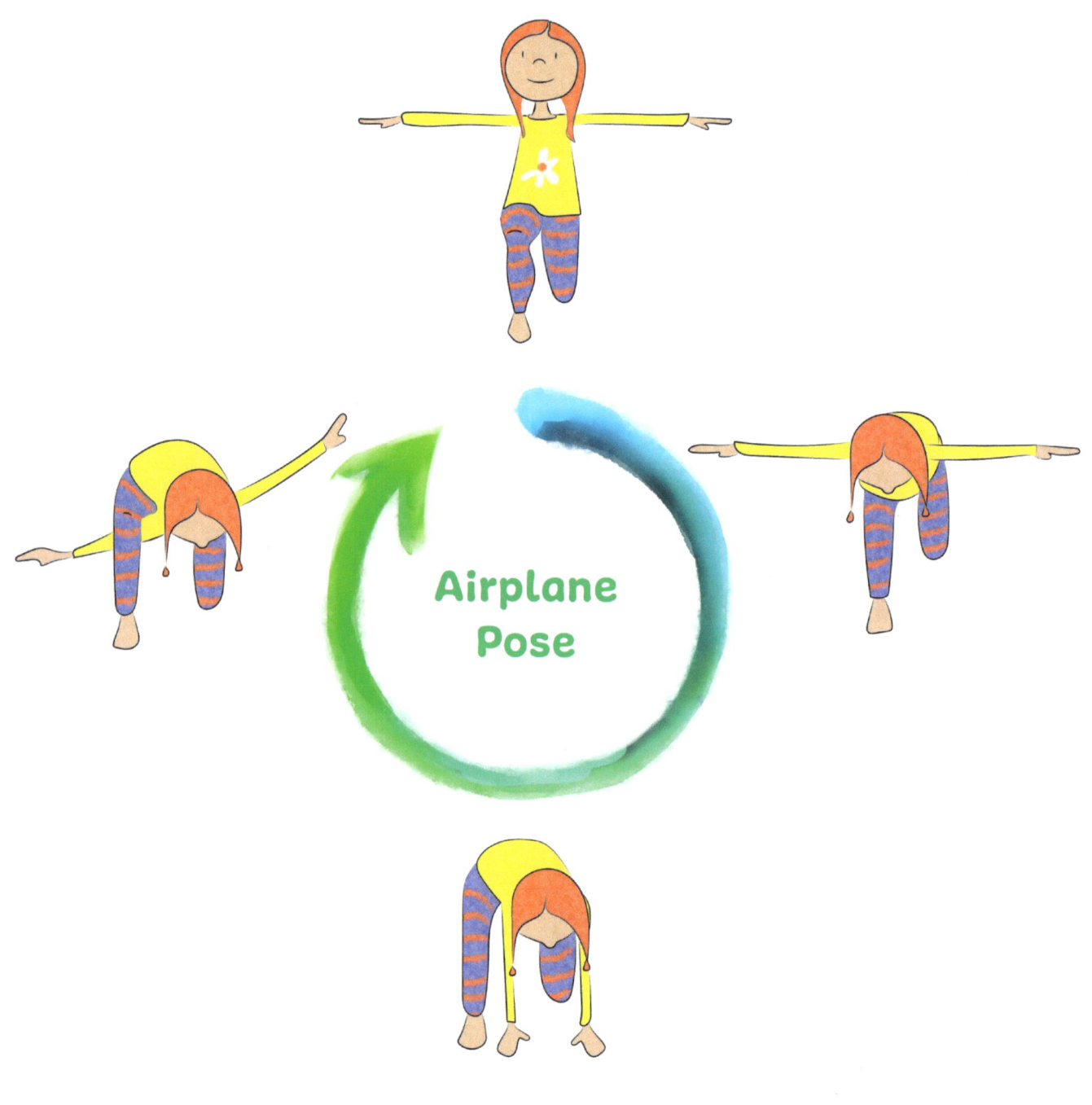

Airplane
Pose

16

Airplane Pose

Inhale, bring your arms out to the side.

Exhale, step one foot forward in lunge.

Inhale, place back knee on the ground.

Inhale, lay your chest on top of your front thigh.

Bring your arms out to the side.

Breathe deeply in the pose.

Inhale deeply.

Exhale fully.

Inhale all the way.

Exhale, let all your breath out.

Return to standing and try this pose on the other leg.

"Whooaa. The trees look super cool from up here," says Danny.

"Trees produce oxygen and help keep our air clean," says Freddy.

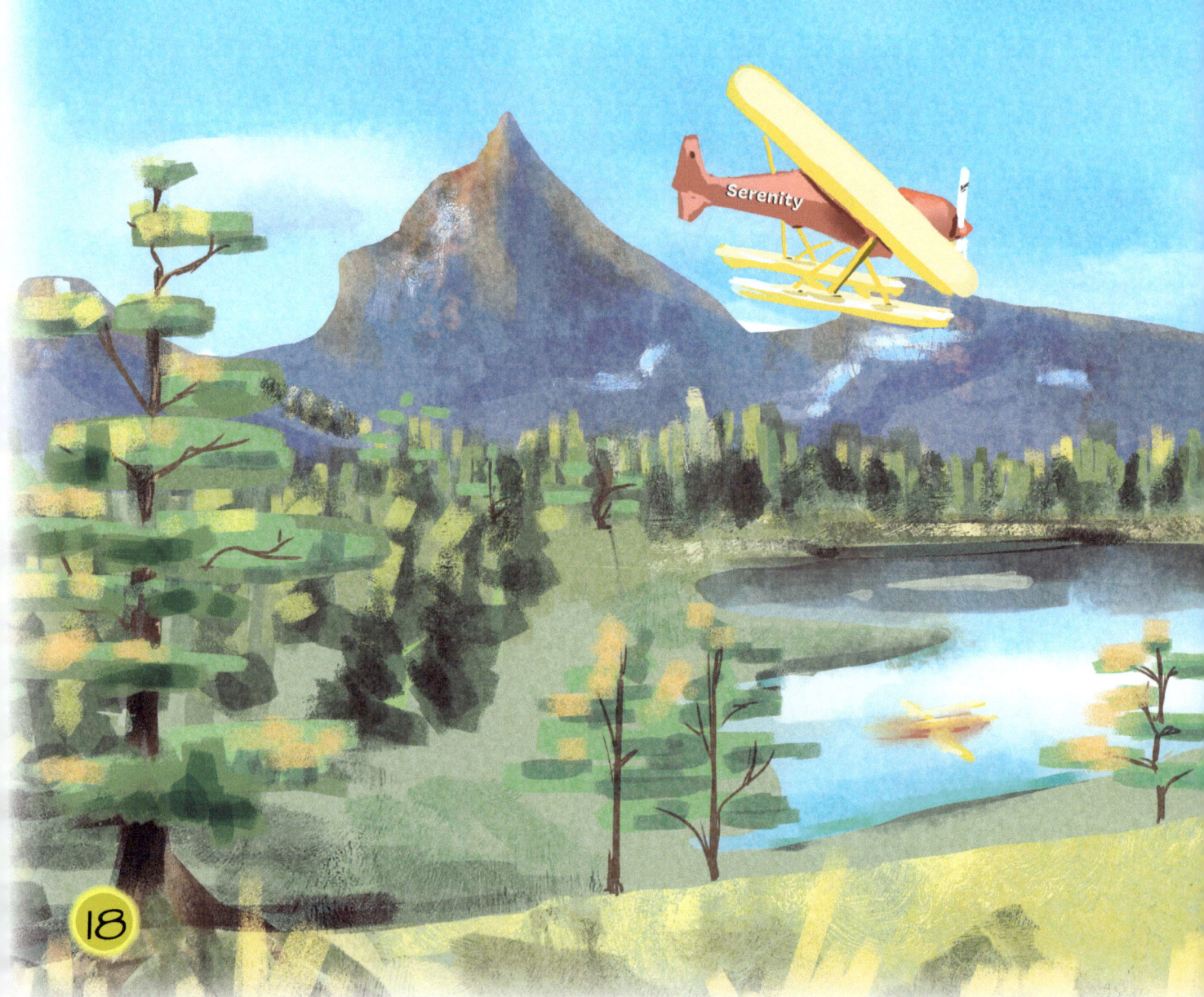

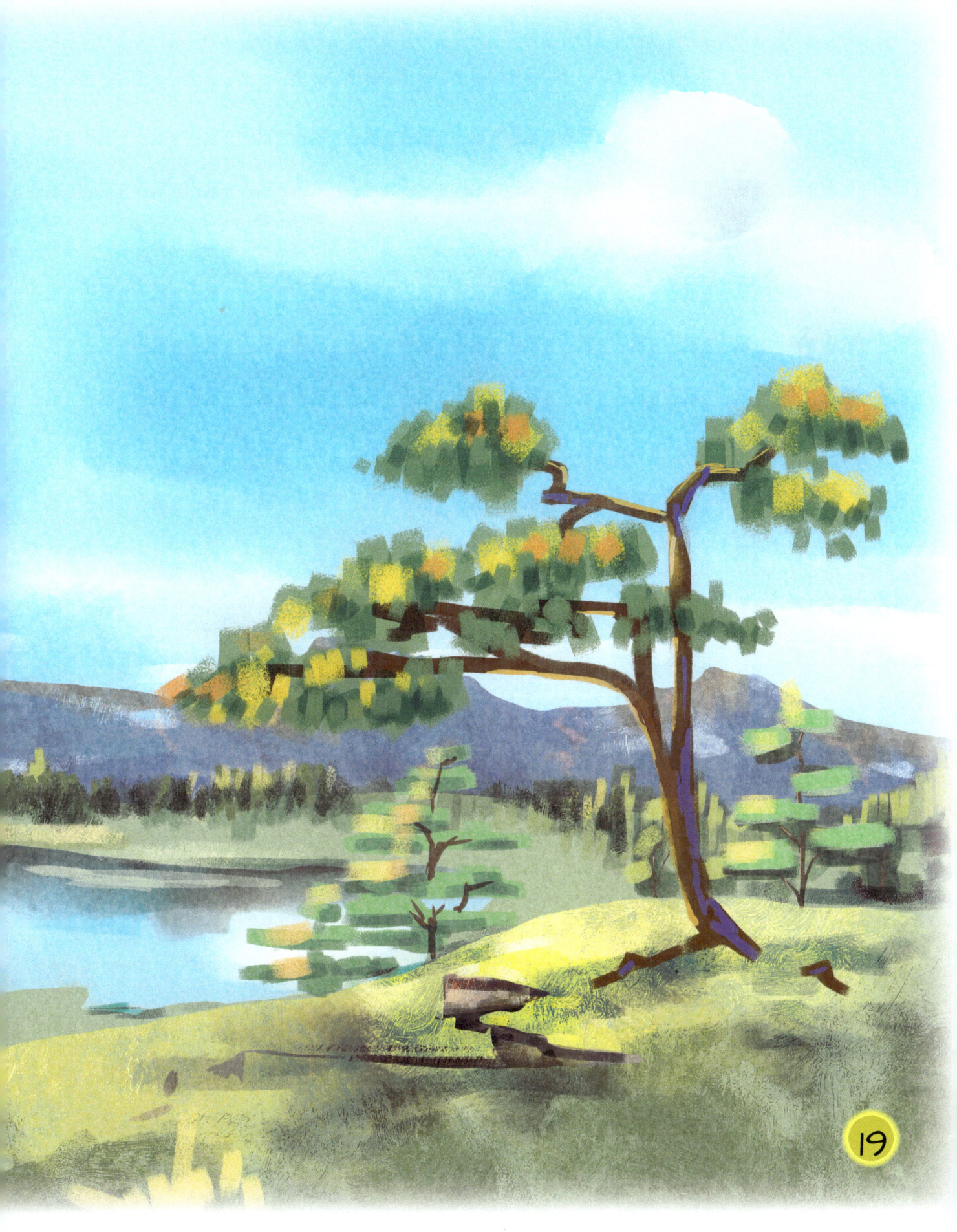

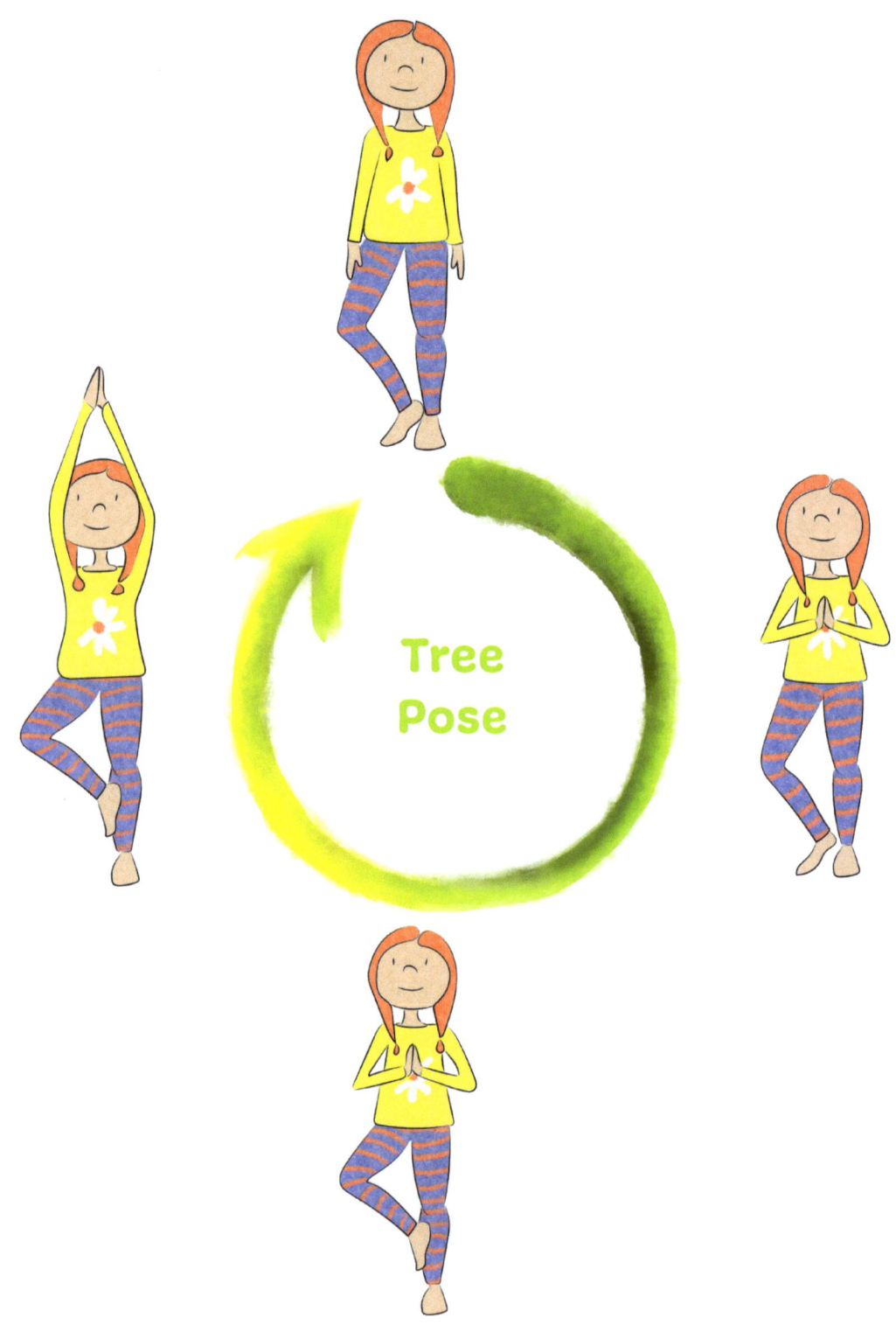

Tree
Pose

Tree Pose

Inhale, place your heel on the inside of your other ankle.

Exhale, bring your hands together in a triangle in front of your heart.

Look at something still in front of you.

Balancing is easier when your eyes are looking at one thing.

Inhale deeply, exhale fully. Keep your body still.

If you feel balanced, slide your foot up your calf.

Try bringing your hands above your head, palms together.

Keep your eyes focused on something small and still.

Breathe deeply.

Pretend you are a tree, with roots deep in the ground.

And branches reaching up to the sky!

Return to standing and try this pose again on the other leg.

"There's Eileen the Eagle," says Freddy.

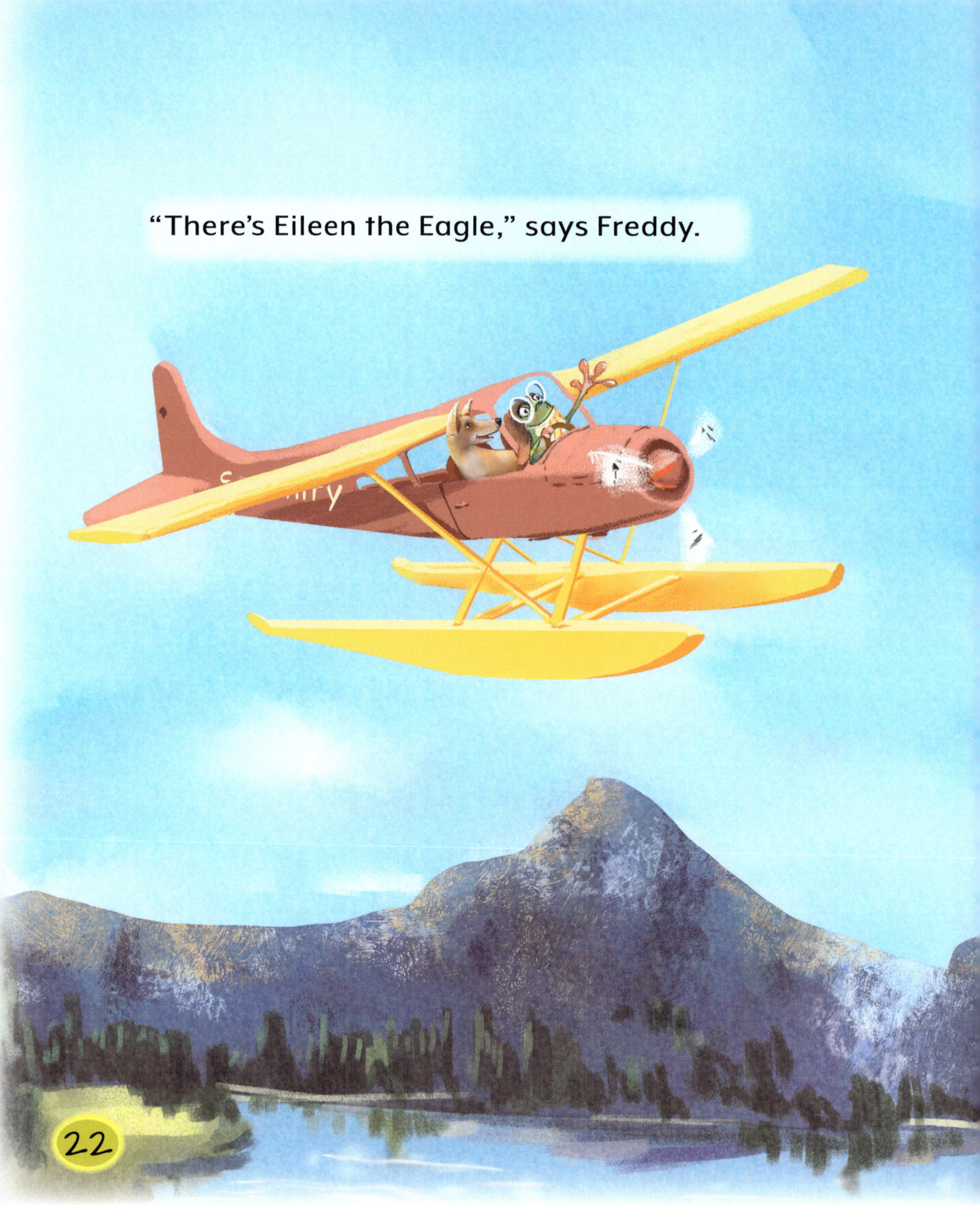

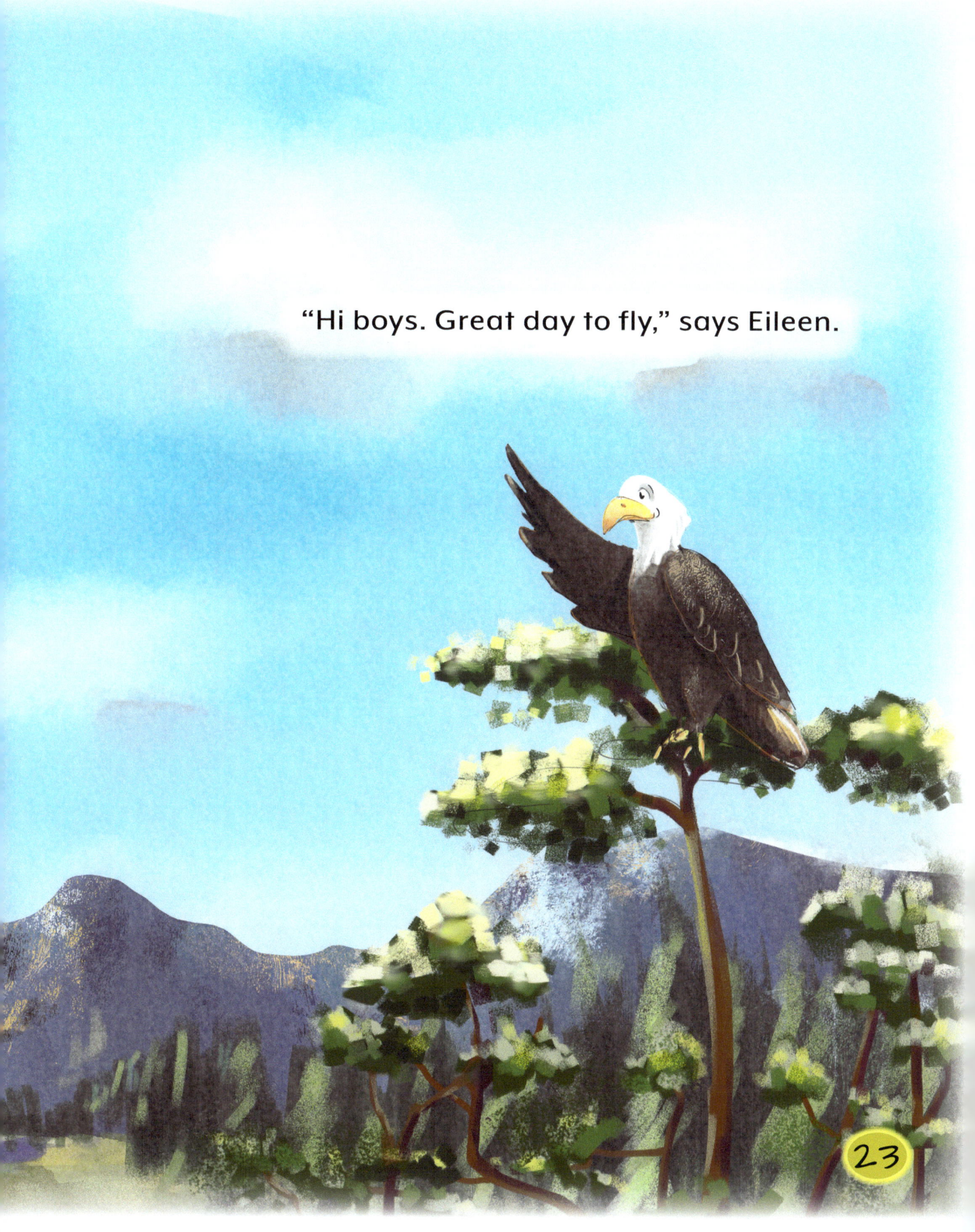

"Hi boys. Great day to fly," says Eileen.

23

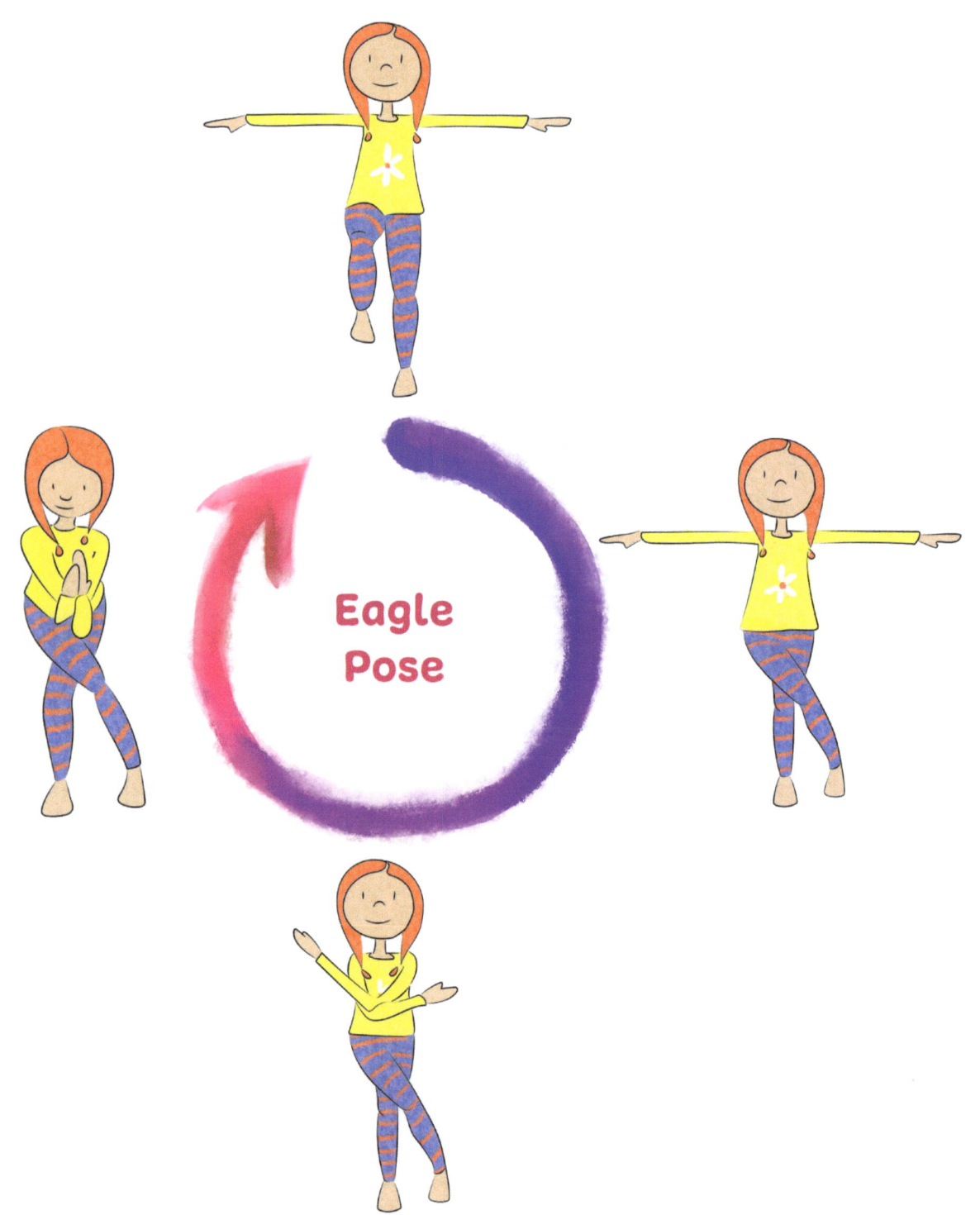

Eagle
Pose

Eagle Pose

From standing, lift one foot off the floor.

Place that knee on top of the other.

Bring your toe to the floor and arms out to the side.

Now cross one elbow on top of the other.

Breathe deeply.

To balance, look at something still in front of you.

Try not to move your eyes as you breathe deeply in and out.

Keeping your eyes on one point is called 'gaze'.

Breathe in deeply, and breathe out fully.

Come out of the pose after a few deep breaths.

Return to standing and try this pose on the other leg.

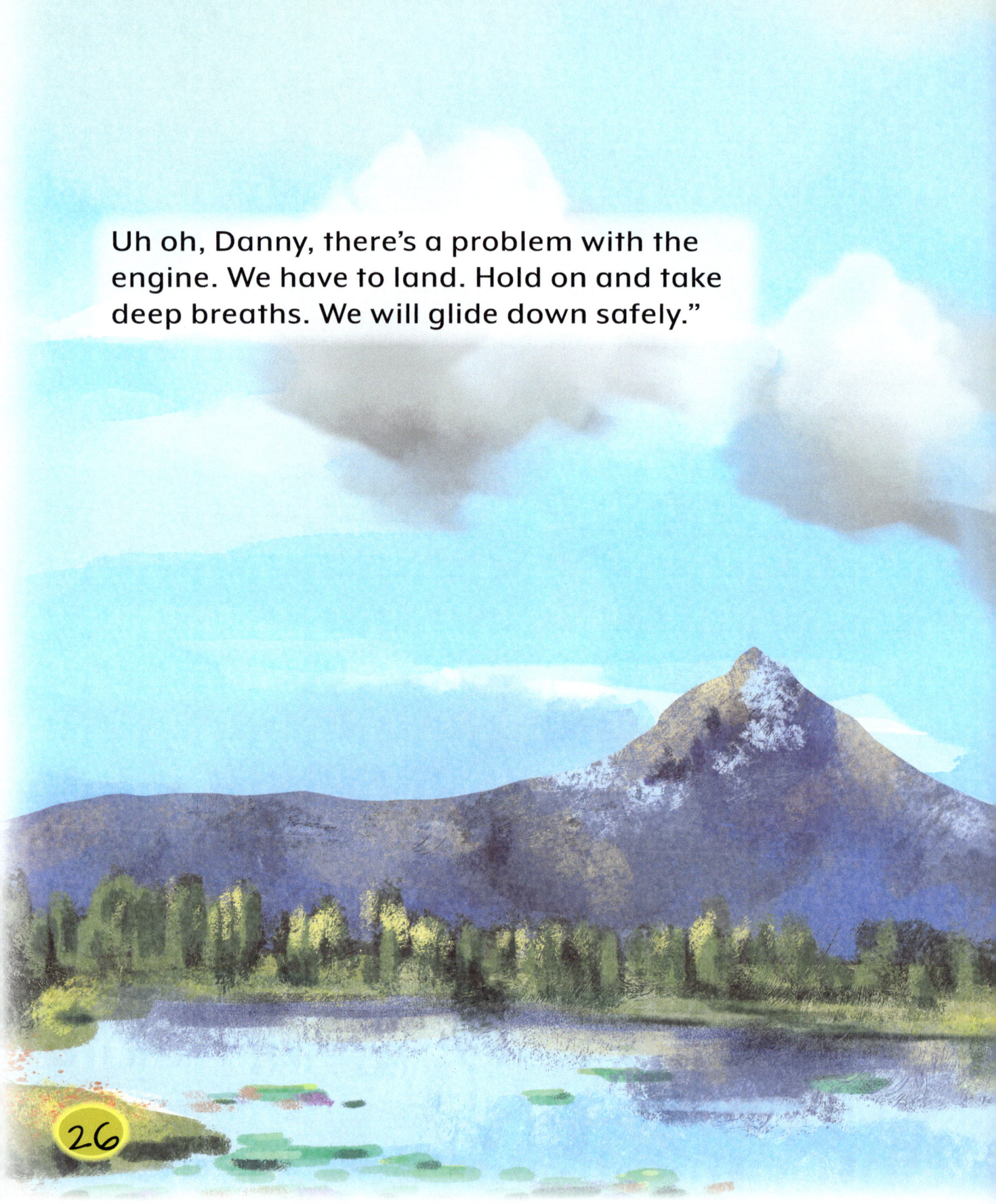

Uh oh, Danny, there's a problem with the engine. We have to land. Hold on and take deep breaths. We will glide down safely."

26

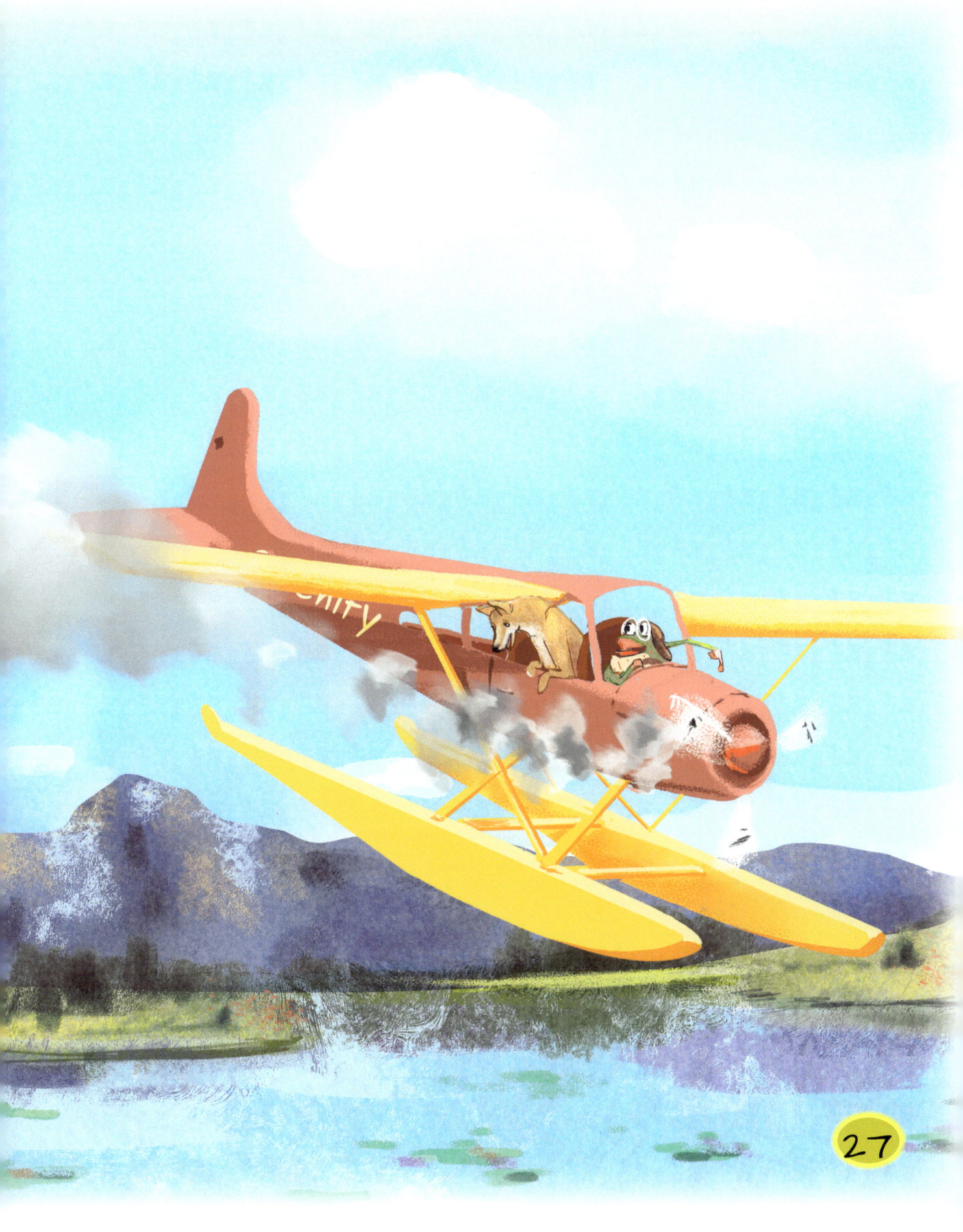

27

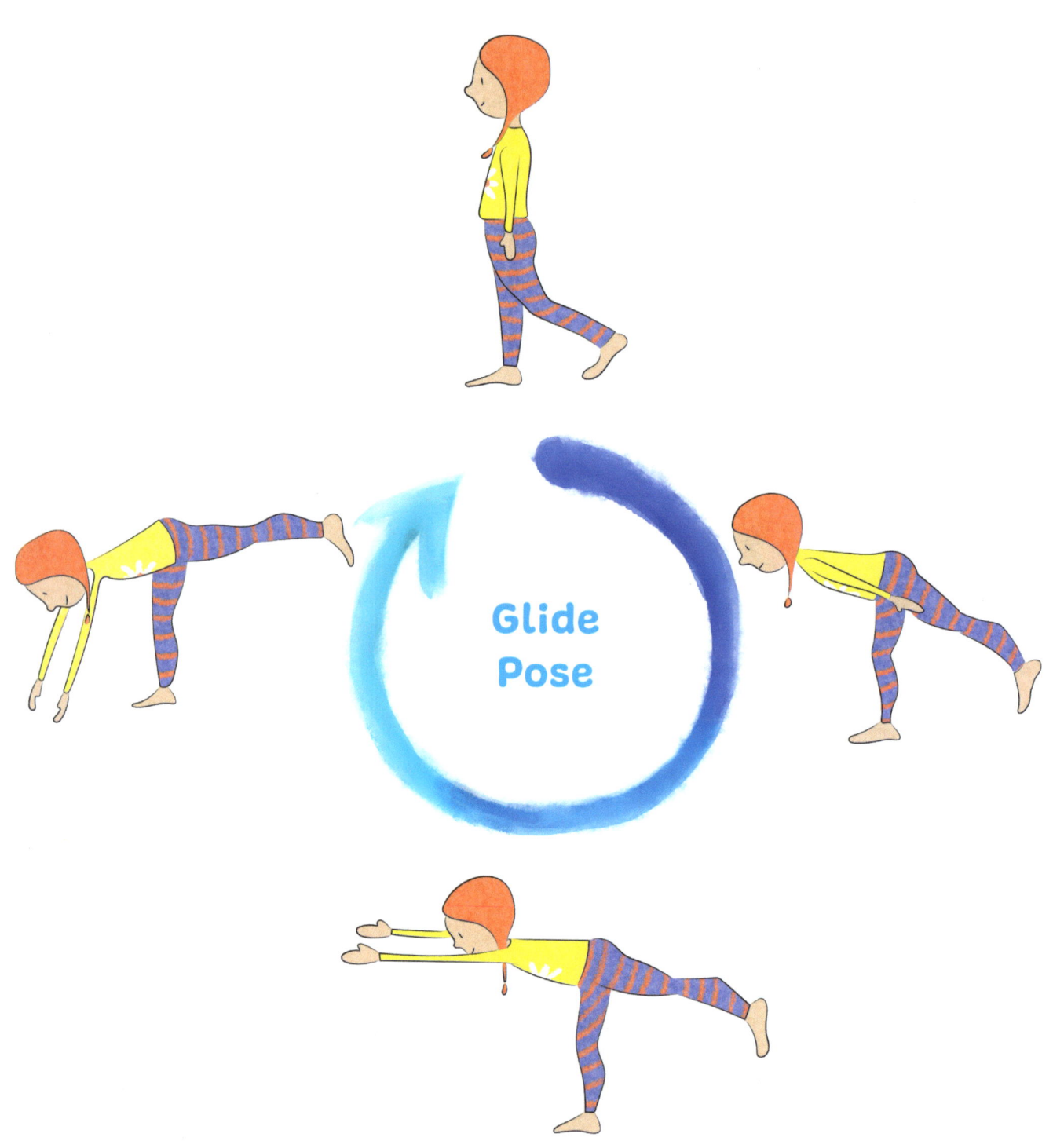

Glide
Pose

Glide Pose

Begin by gazing at a point on the ground in front of you.

Inhale and slide one foot behind you.

Exhale, tilt forward and bring your hands in front of you.
Try not to look around the room.

Inhale and gently glide your hands down toward the floor.
Bend your knees if needed.

Keep your eyes gazed and breath flowing deeply.

Return to standing and try this pose on the other leg.

"Freddy, where are we?" says Danny. "How will we find our way back to Pondering Pond?"

"Hmmm, ribitt." says Freddy. "Let me have a look around."

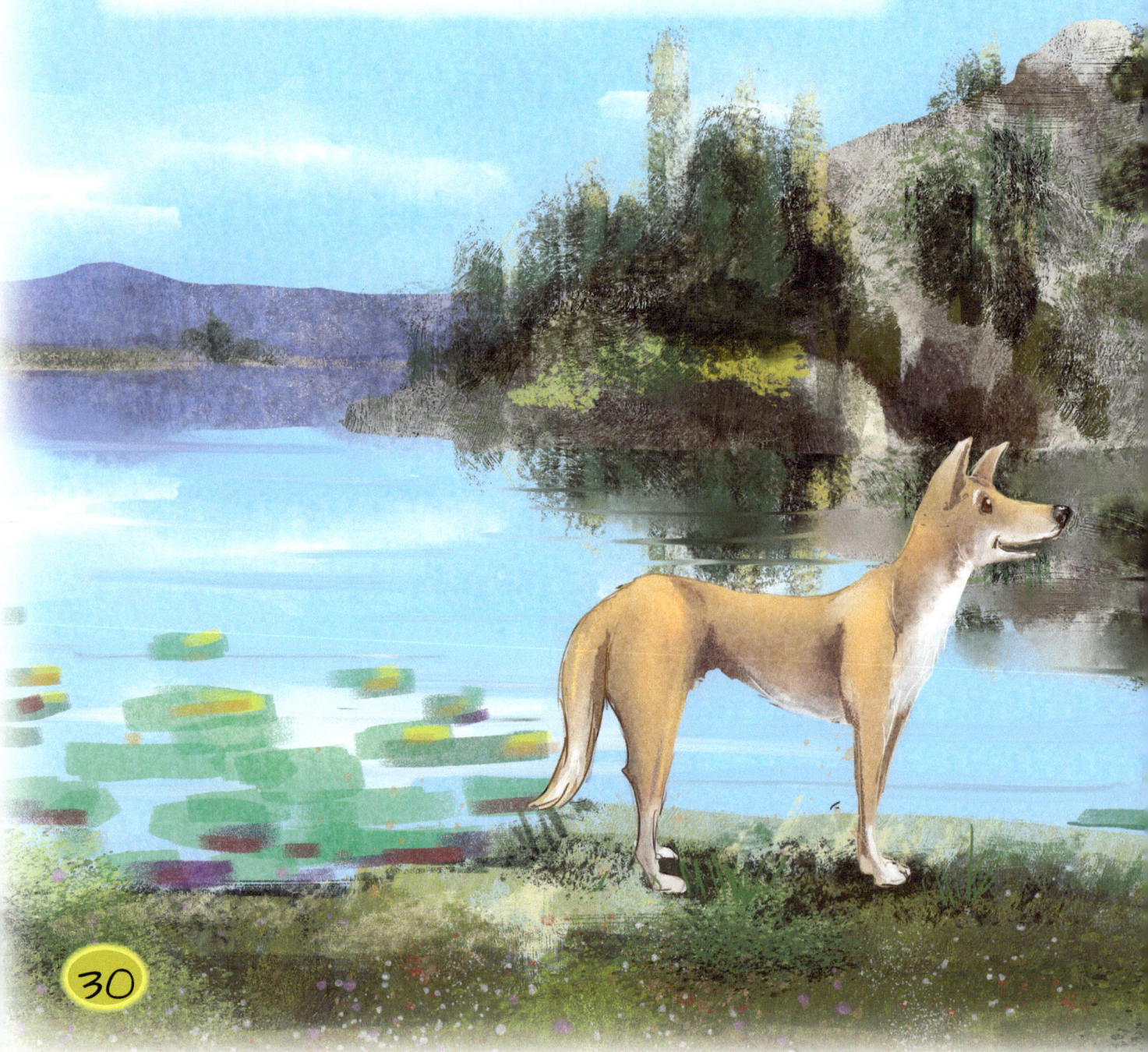

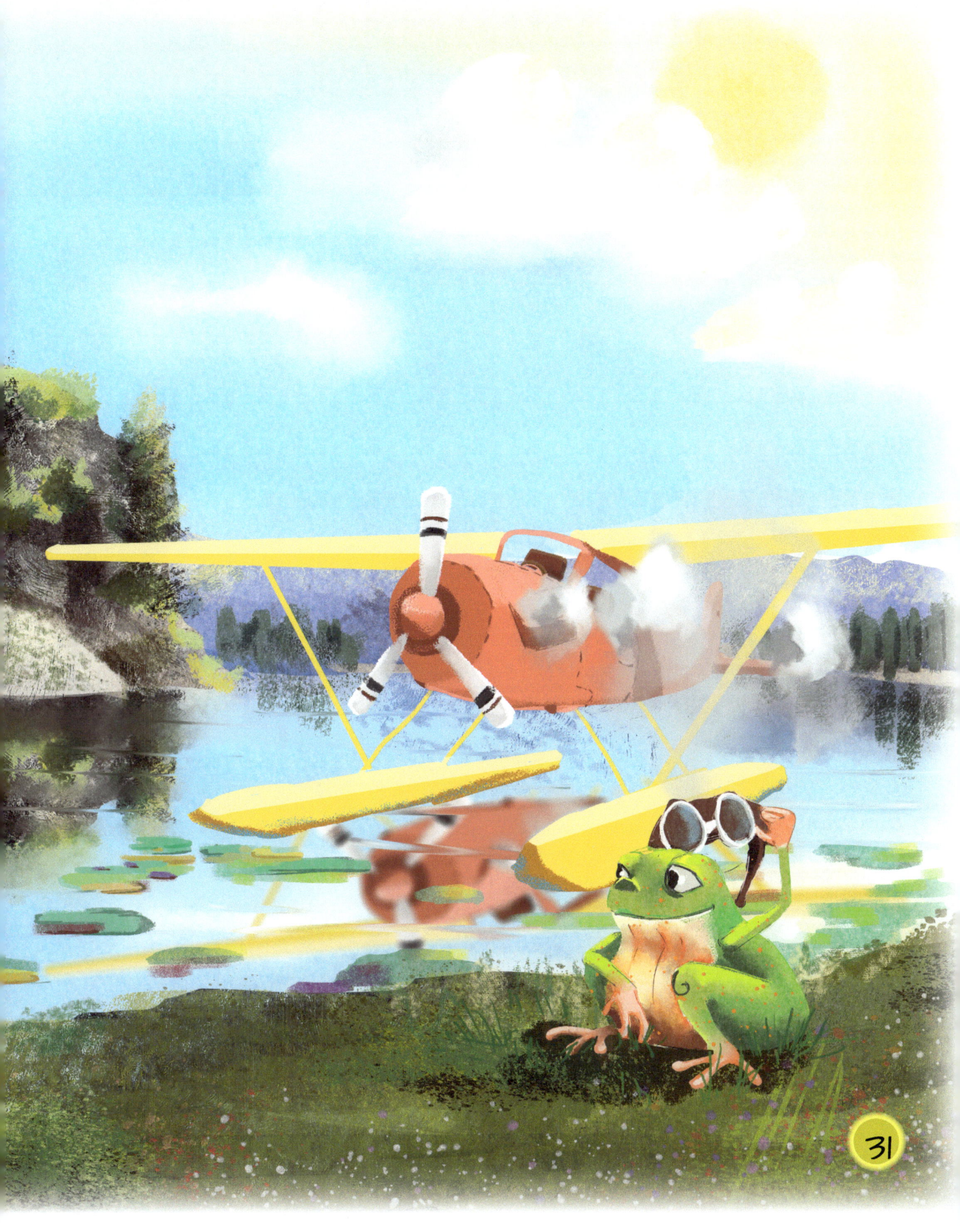

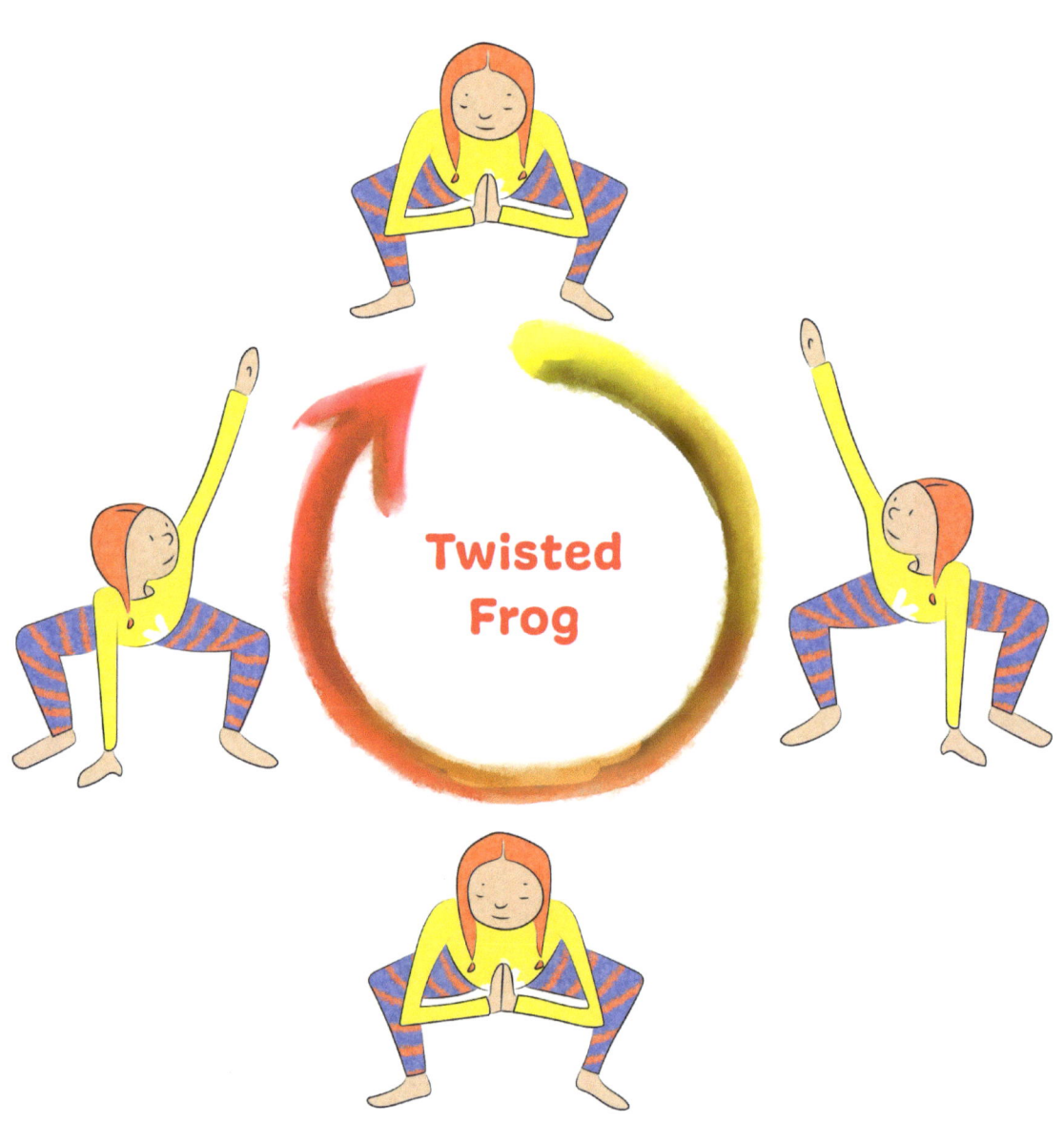

Twisted Frog

Twisted Frog

Stand with your feet wider than your hips.
Squat down and try to keep your feet flat on the floor.

Place your palms together in front of your heart.
Breathe deeply and enjoy the stretch.

Then bring one hand to the ground in front of you.
Lift the other hand up in the air. Breathe deeply in
this twist. Gaze at your thumb in the air.
Stay here for a few deep breaths.
Return to center with palms together at your heart.

Repeat by bringing the other hand flat on the ground in front of you.
Lift the other arm in the air.
Breathe deeply in and out a few times!

Return to a comfortable seated position.

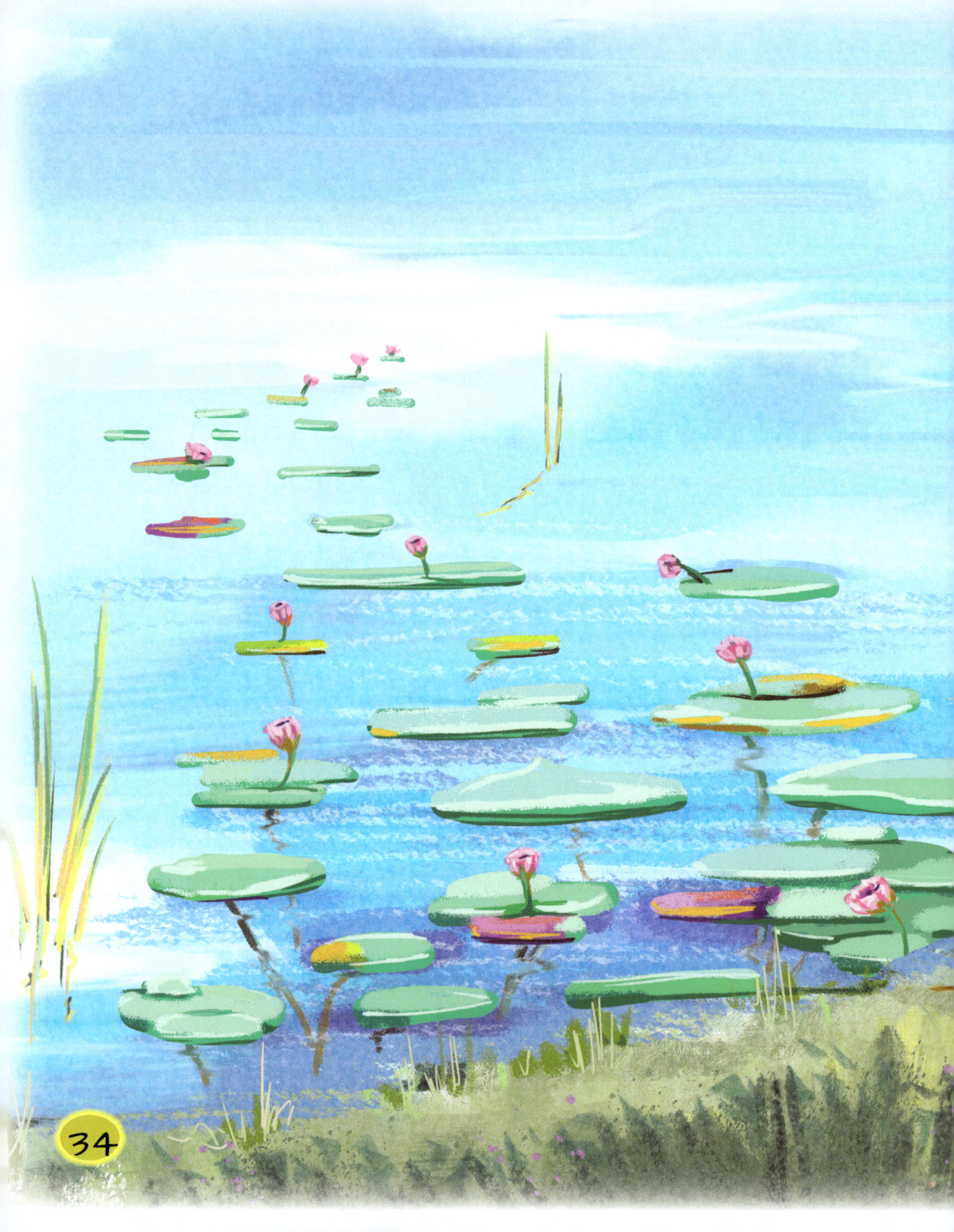

"Look at the lily pads. They are showing us the way home," says Freddy. If we leap from one to the next, they will guide us."

"So cool! This day keeps getting better," says Danny.

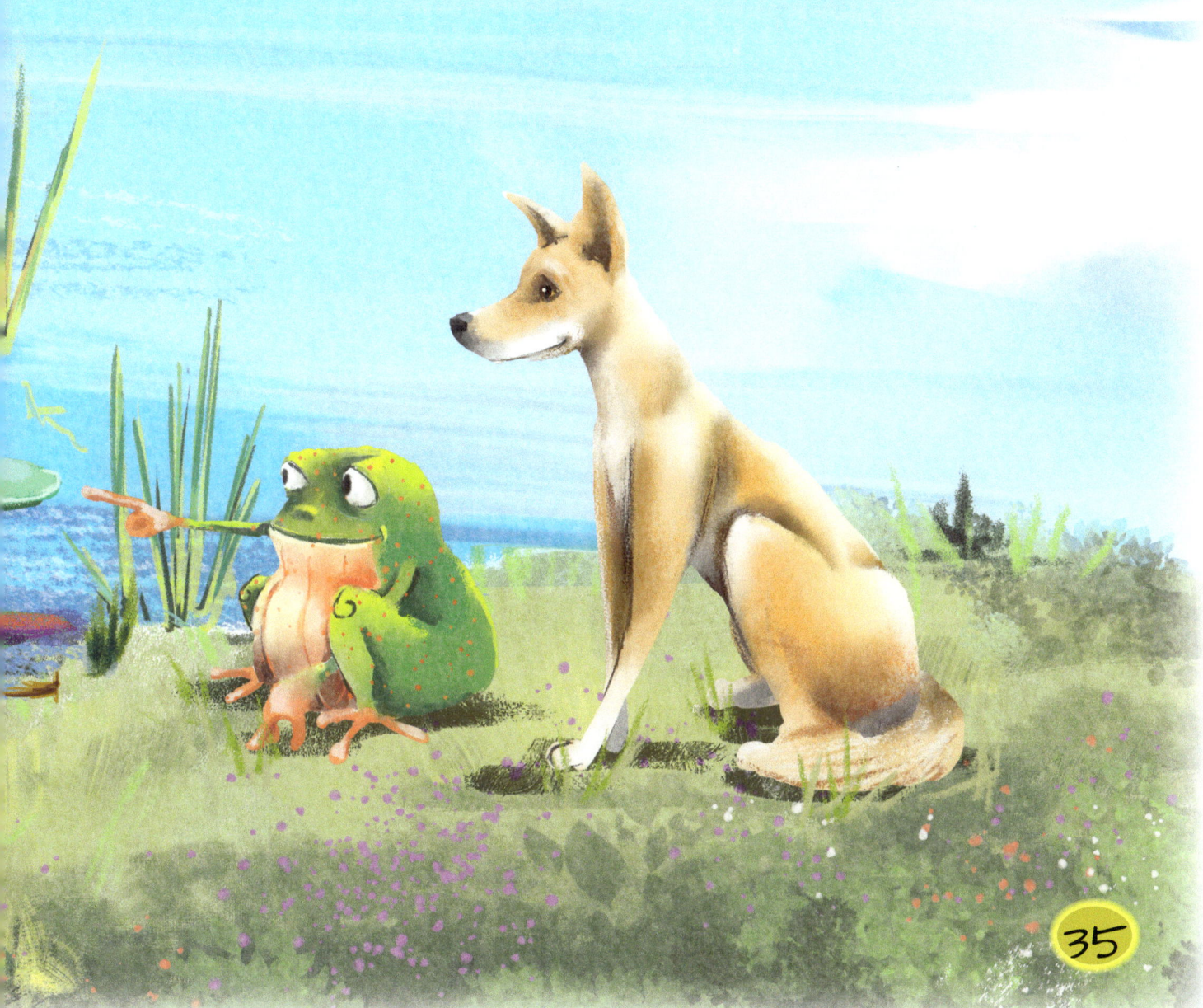

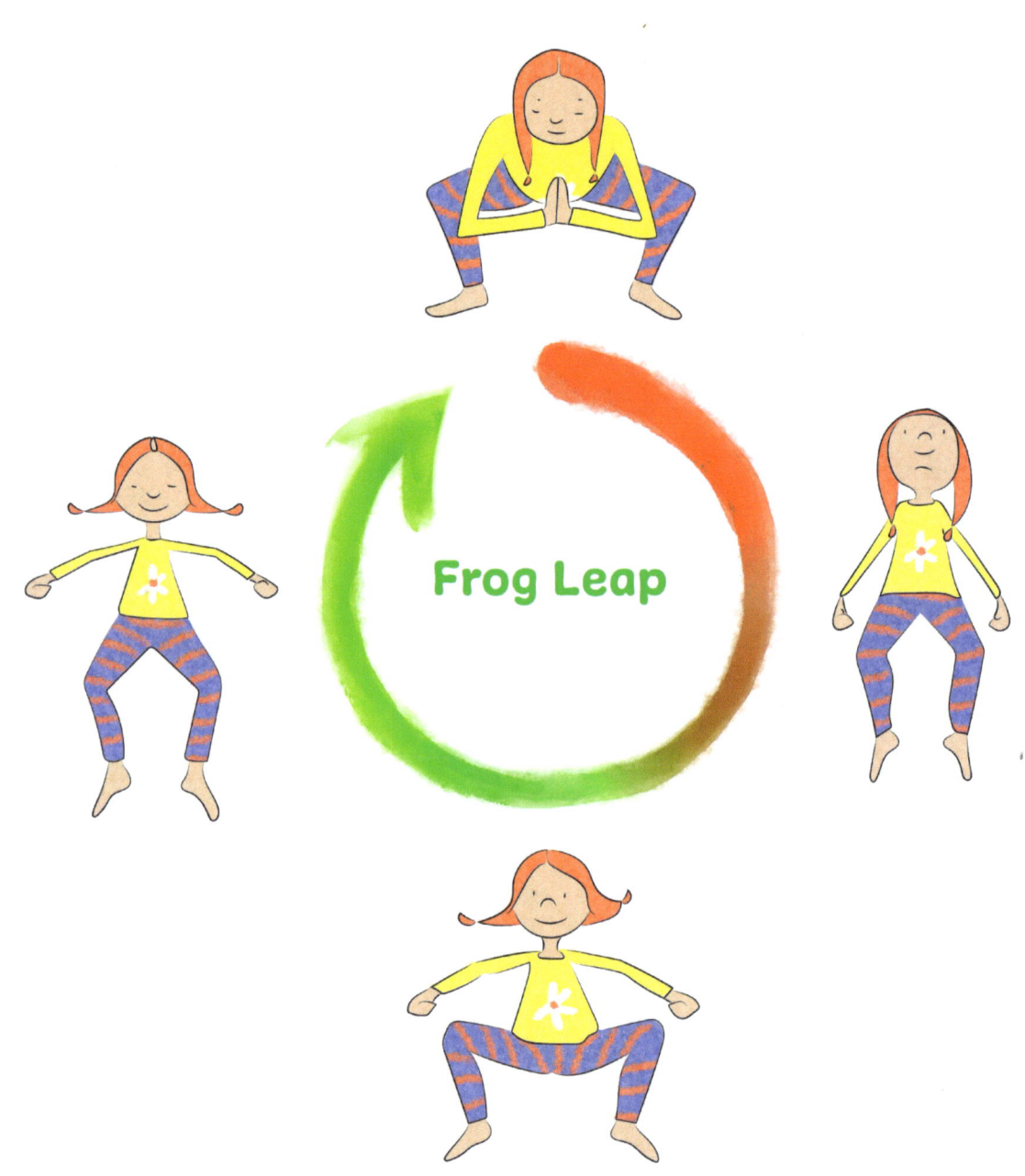

Frog Leap

Frog Leap

Begin in frog pose.

Hands together and feet flat on the ground.

Without moving forward or backward, leap straight up in the air.

When you leap, try to bring your knees up to your ears.

Land gently and quietly.

Try doing 8 frog leaps.

Rest, and repeat 8 more frog leaps if you can!

Remember to leap straight up.

Bring your knees up as high as you can.

When you are finished, sit down in a cross legged position.

Place your palms on your knees.

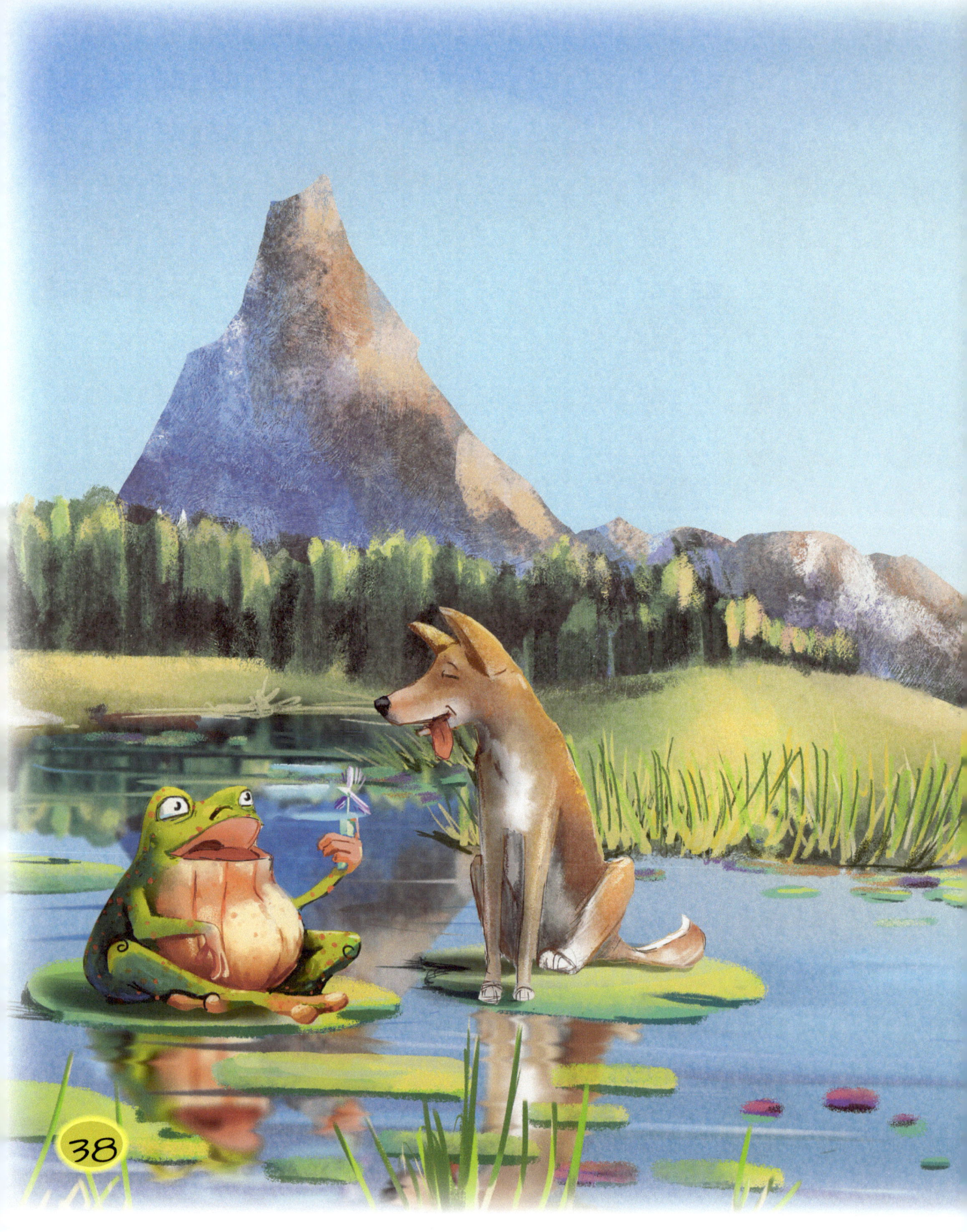

"What a leaping journey, but we made it back to Pondering Pond," says Freddy. Be still and feel your heart beating Danny, its been working hard with all those leaps."

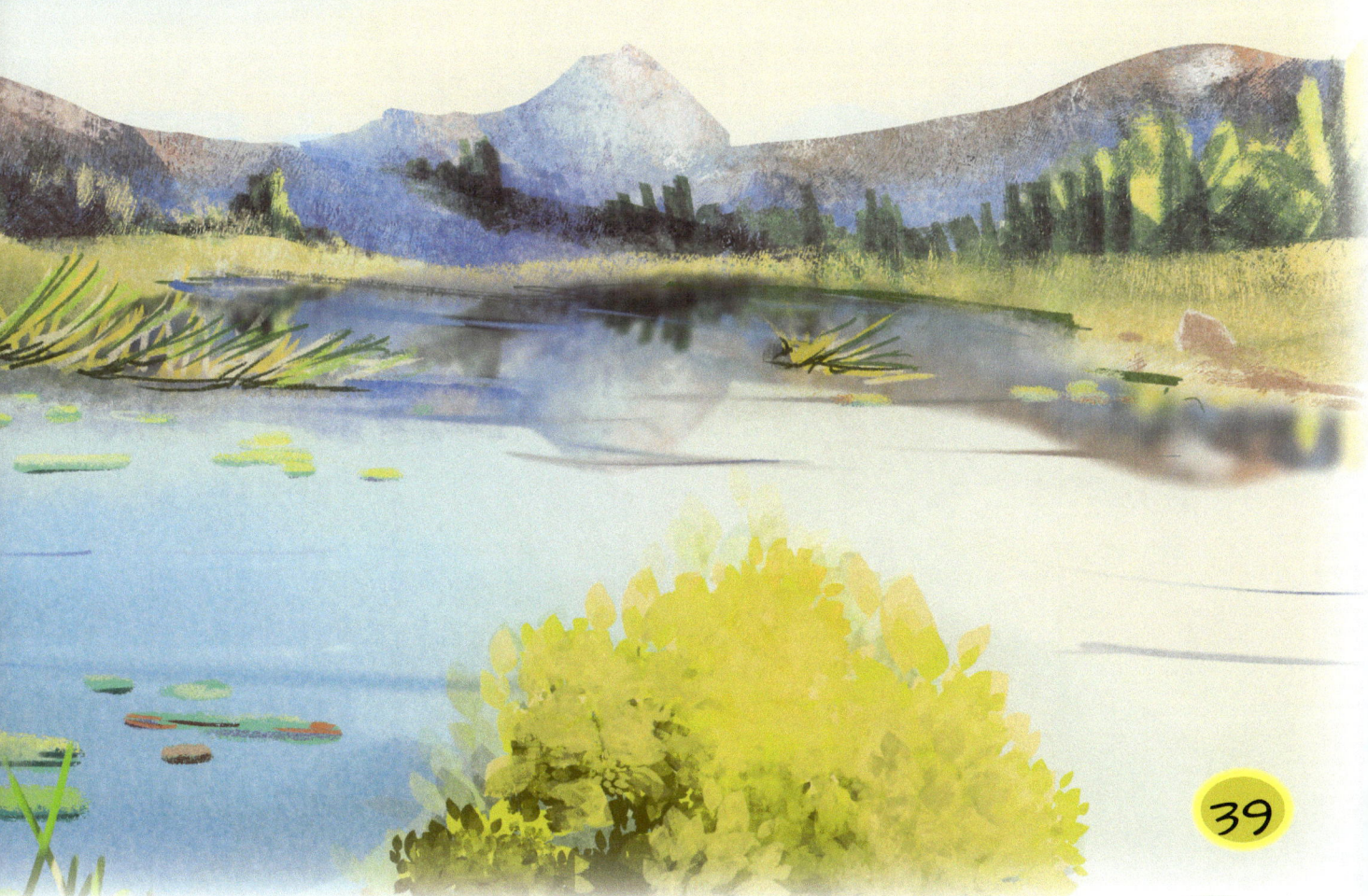

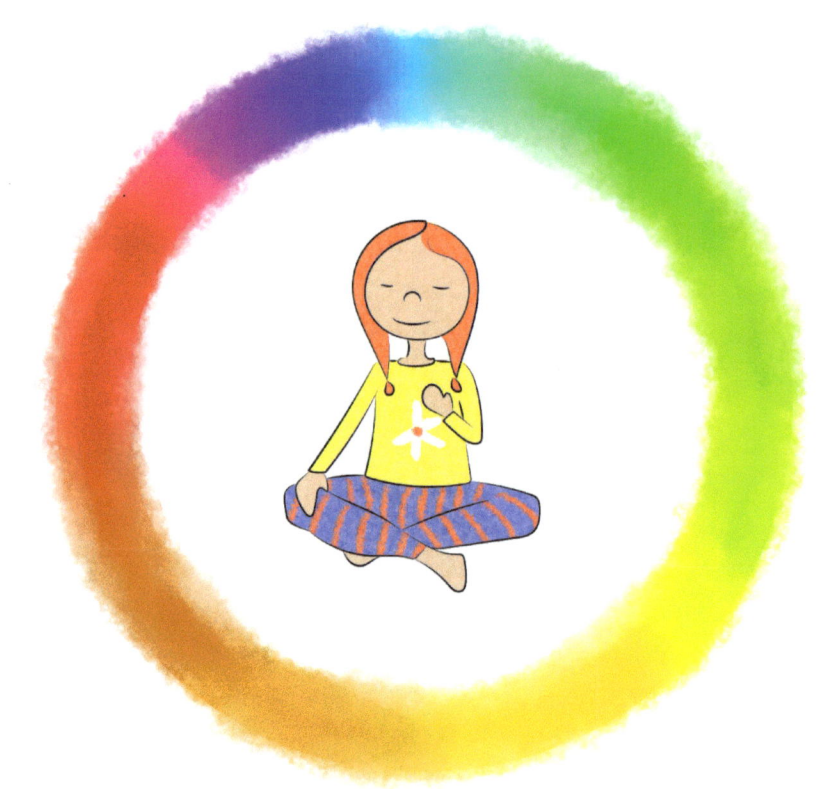

Feel Your Heart

Find a comfortable seated position.

Place your right hand near your heart and left hand on your knee.

Close your eyes. Feel your heart beating.

Is it beating quickly?

Try to be still, without any movement in your body.

Can you feel your heart slowing down as you relax?

Keep your eyes closed.

Bring all of your attention to your heart.

It works hard to keep you alive.

With your hand on your heart, whisper, "Thank you heart."

Stay in this pose as long as you like.

When you are finished, stay seated and open your eyes.

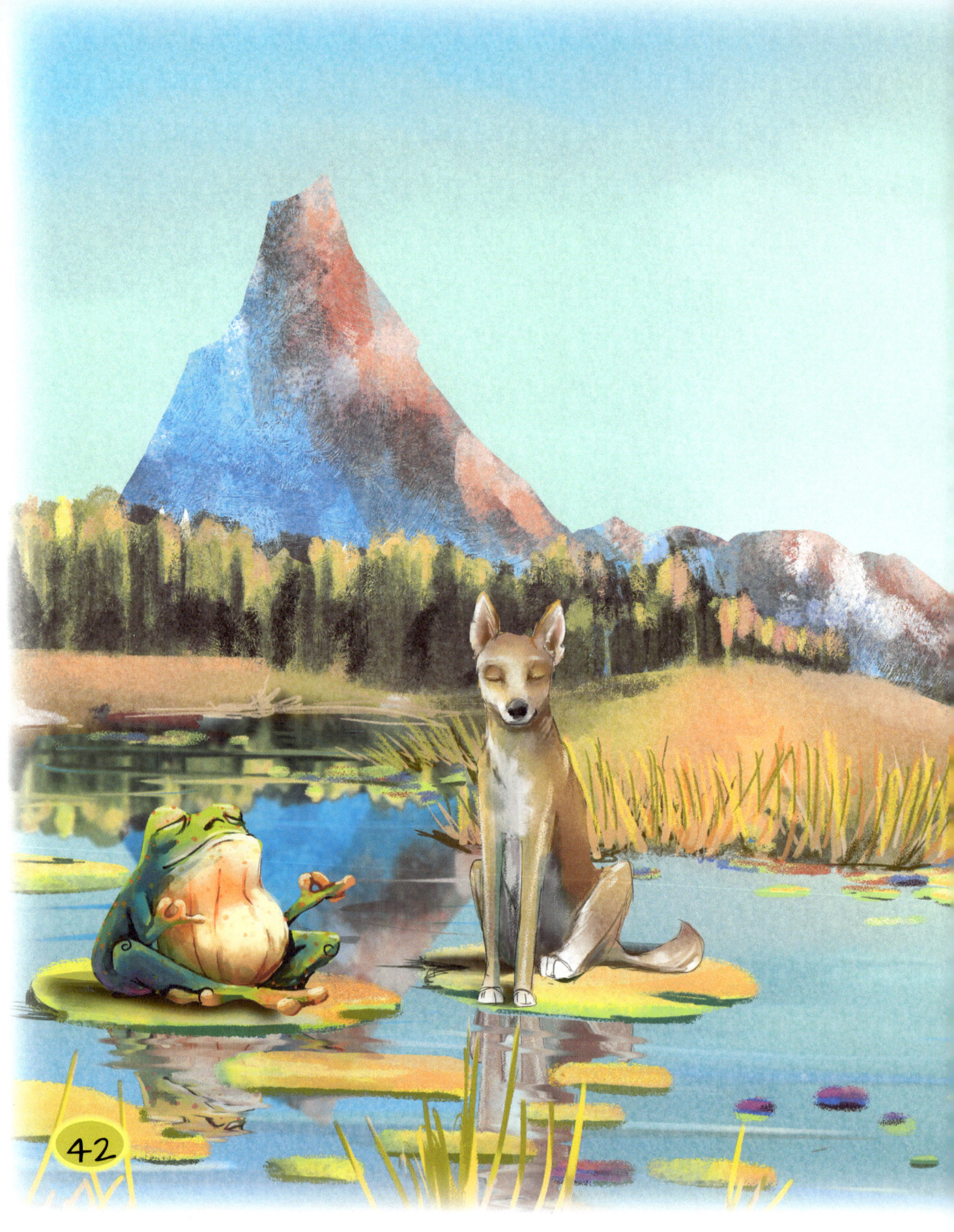

"Danny, let's try an experiment," says Freddy.

"Breathe in deeply through your nose and feel your breath.

Bring your attention to where your breath goes inside your body."

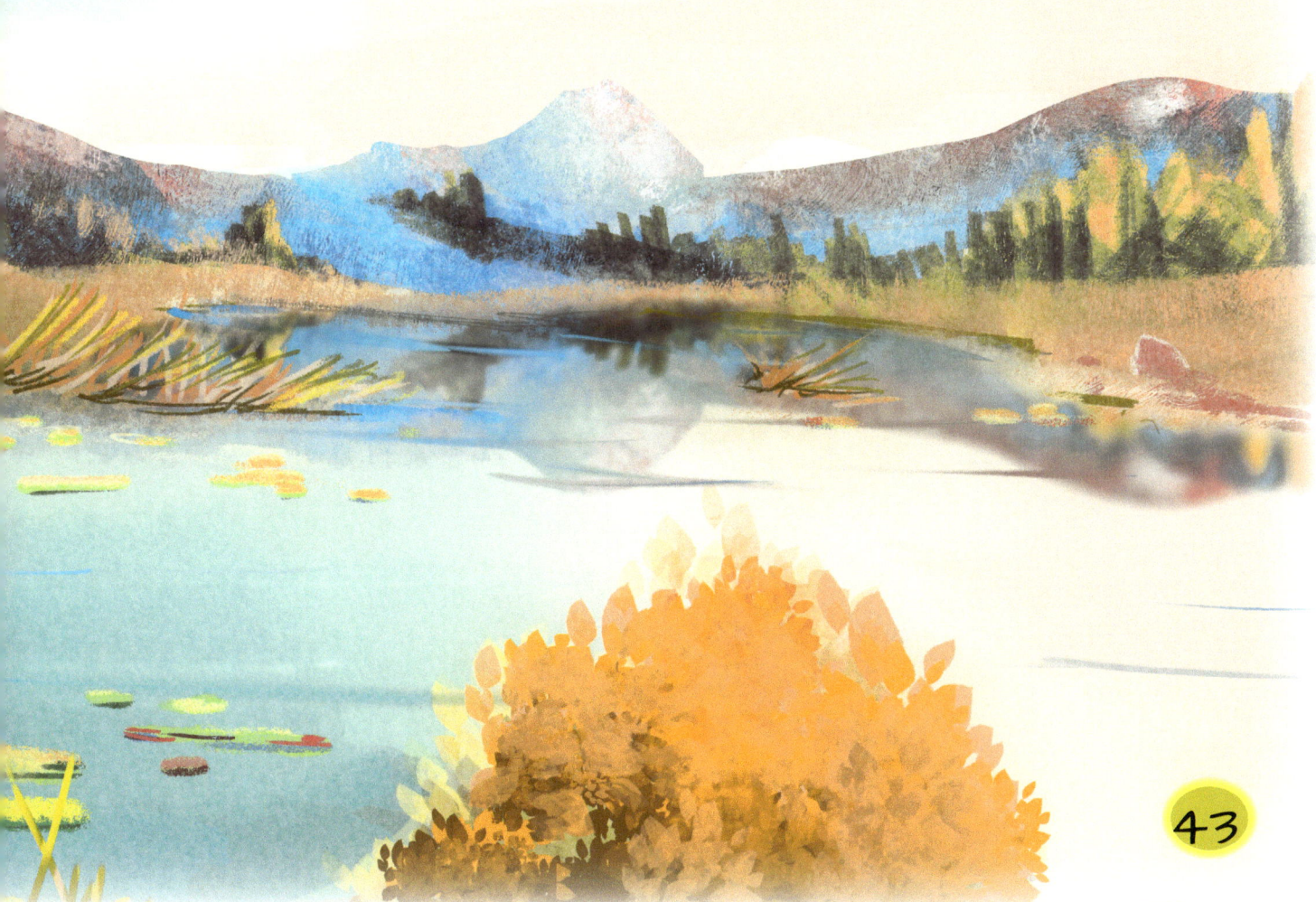

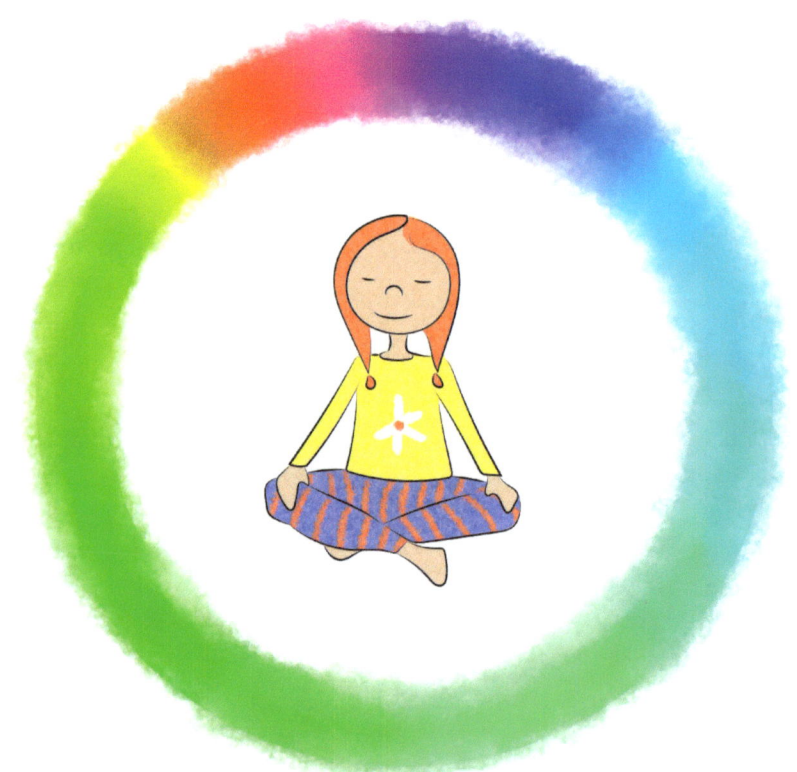

Breath Experiment

Return to stillness with eyes closed.

Bring both hands on top of your knees.

Inhale through your nose deeply.

Exhale through your nose fully.

As you inhale, feel where your breath comes into your body?

As you exhale, feel your breath fill your body.

Stay still and keep your eyes closed.

Relax. Feel your breath as it moves into your body.

Thoughts may come into your mind.

This is natural.

When it happens, return your attention to your breath.

Try this breath experiment for two or three minutes.

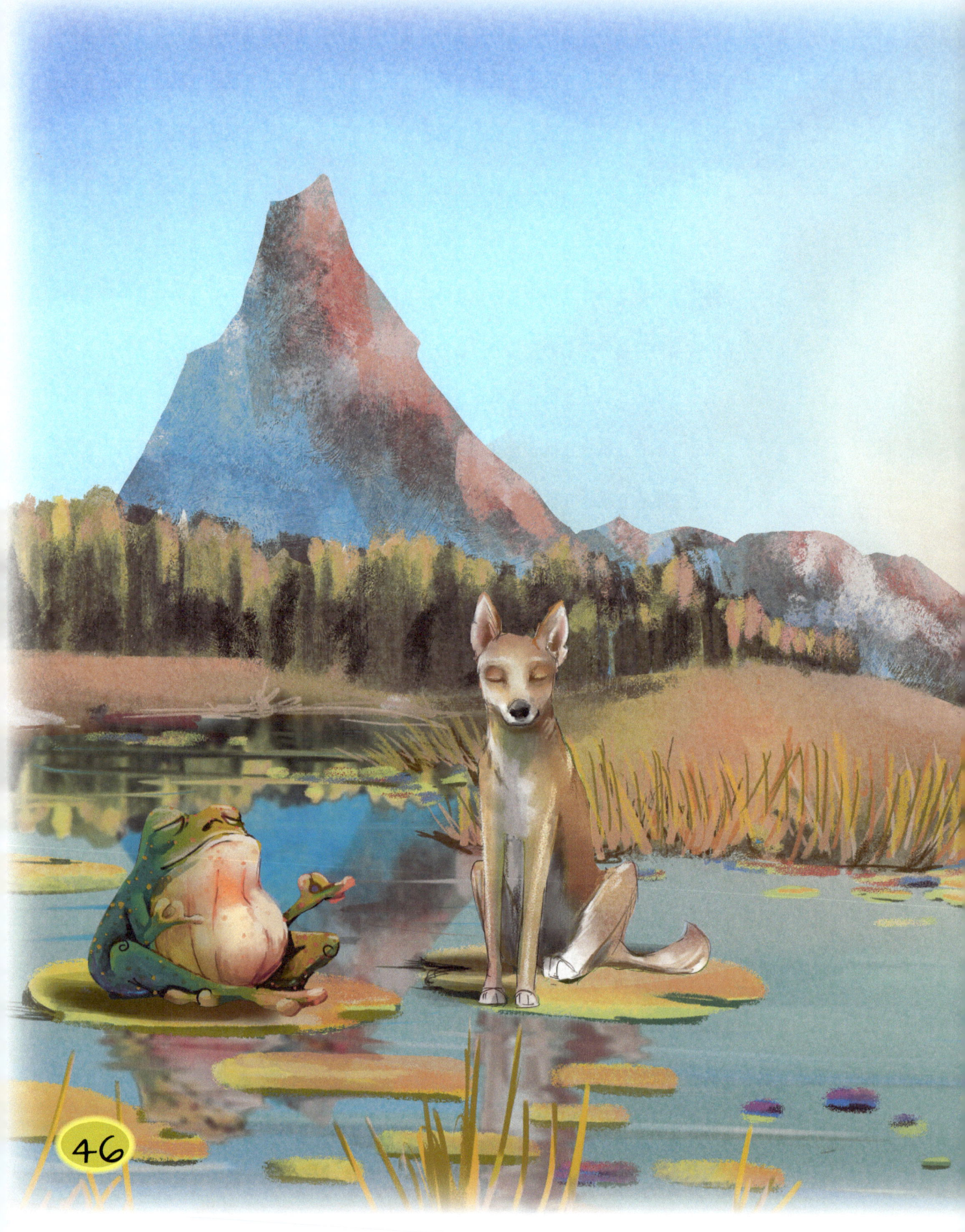

"Danny, you said you did not want to practice meditation because you were afraid you'd make a mistake. But the only mistake you can make in meditation....is not starting"

"Thanks Freddy," says Danny. I am super relaxed. What a great day seeing the world in Serenity."

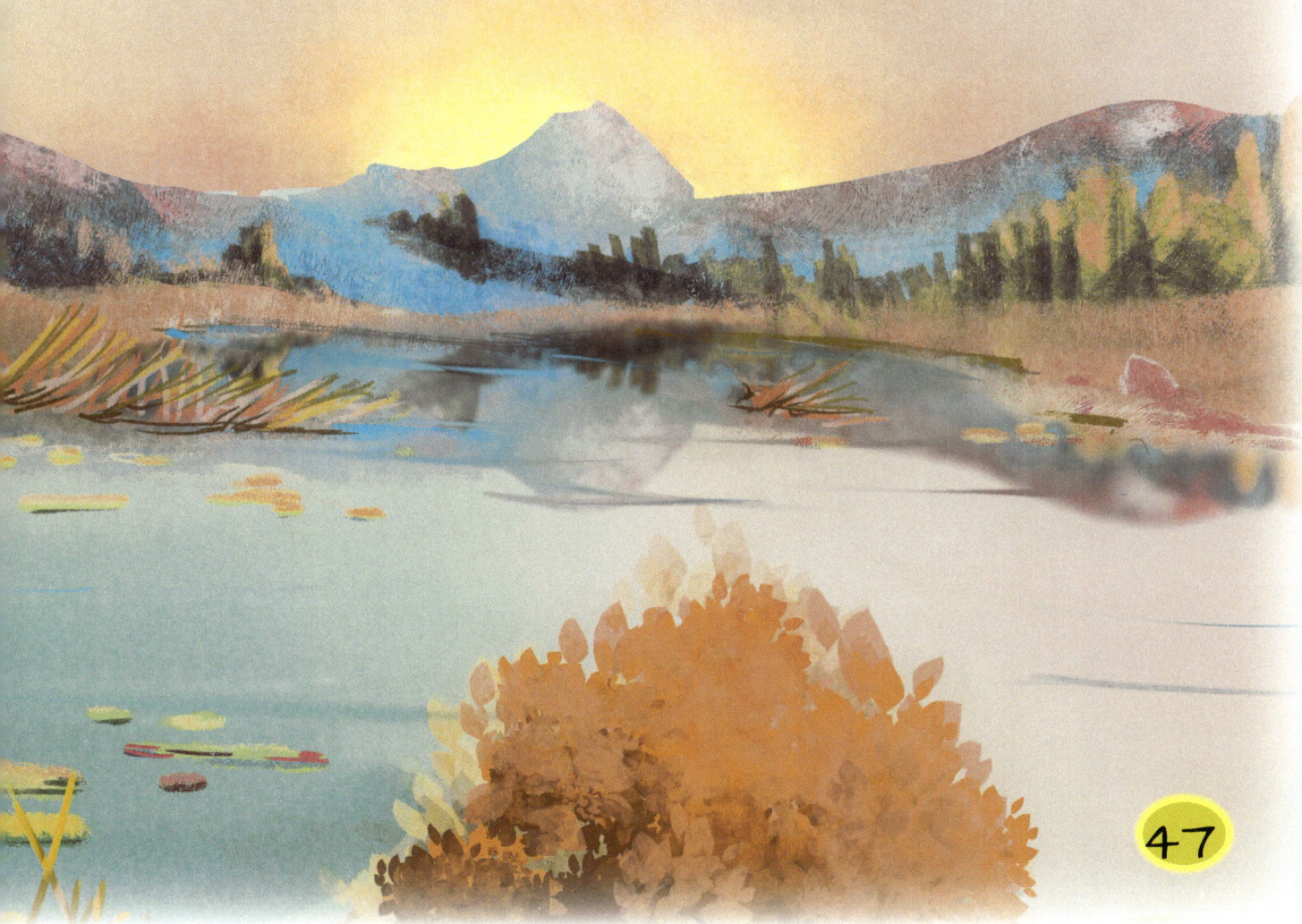

Yoga Poses

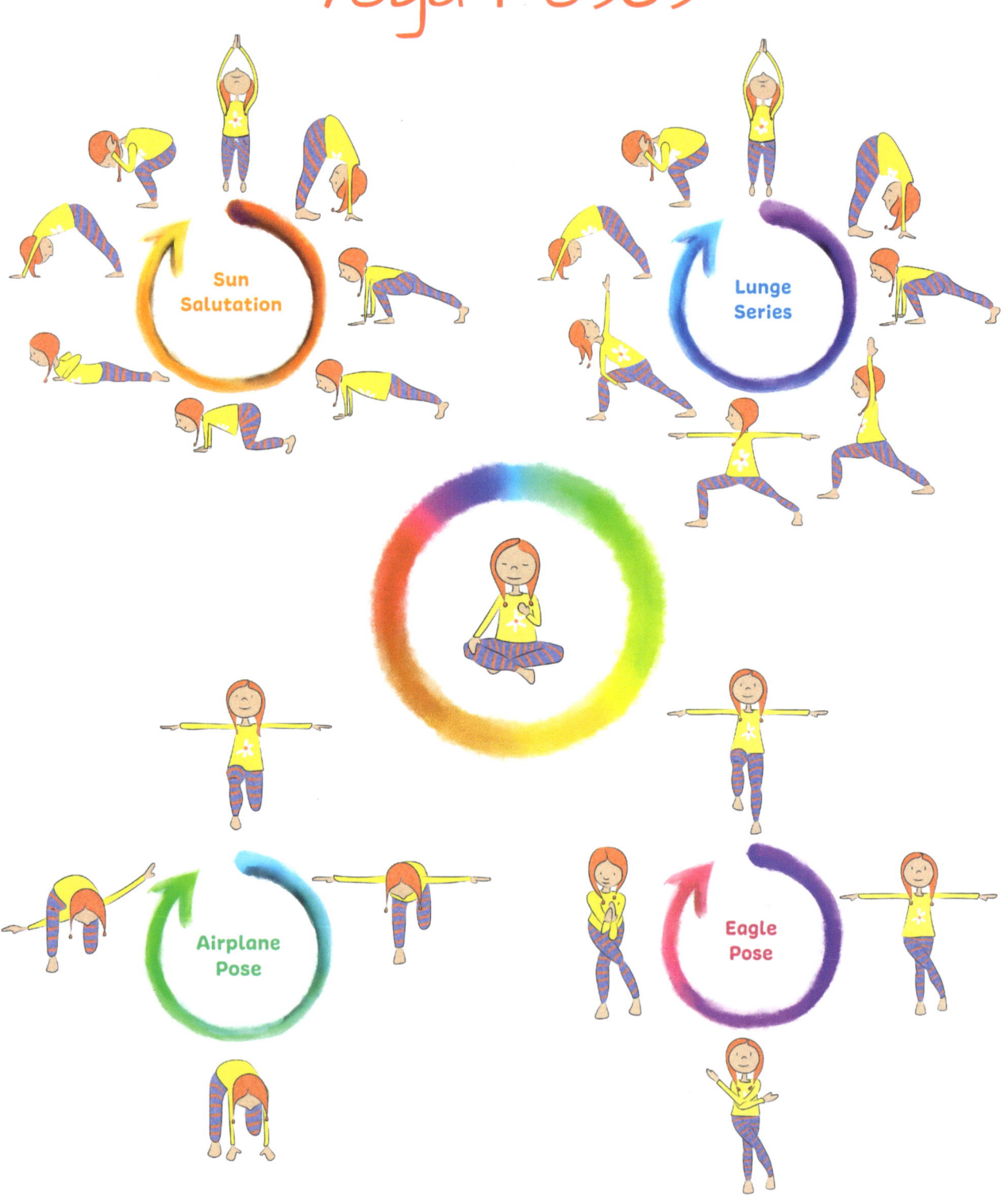

Sun Salutation

Lunge Series

Airplane Pose

Eagle Pose

Yoga Poses

Tree Pose

Twisted Frog

Frog Leap

Glide Pose

YOUR Serenity Matters

Have you ever said "I can't meditate!" Just like Danny in this story knows, sitting still and being calm is difficult. As you and your children begin to practice meditation, it is natural to feel like you can't do it.

But let's explore wise Freddy the Frog's lesson in this book, "the only mistake we can make in meditation is not starting."

In yoga there is a famous story called the Bhagavad Gita where the fate of the unsuccessful meditator is explored. We learn that engaging in calming activities – even if brief – will never be met with anything bad. The very striving for peace and serenity is a most auspicious (or favorable) attempt.

What this means is that any effort aimed at creating calm, whether for yourself or your family, is rewarded. And the key word here is EFFORT, versus success. Whether it's one deep breath in the morning as you help your child get dressed, a few deep breaths in the car on the way to activities, or a brief gratitude moment before a meal, there are no mistakes as you attempt mindful practices.

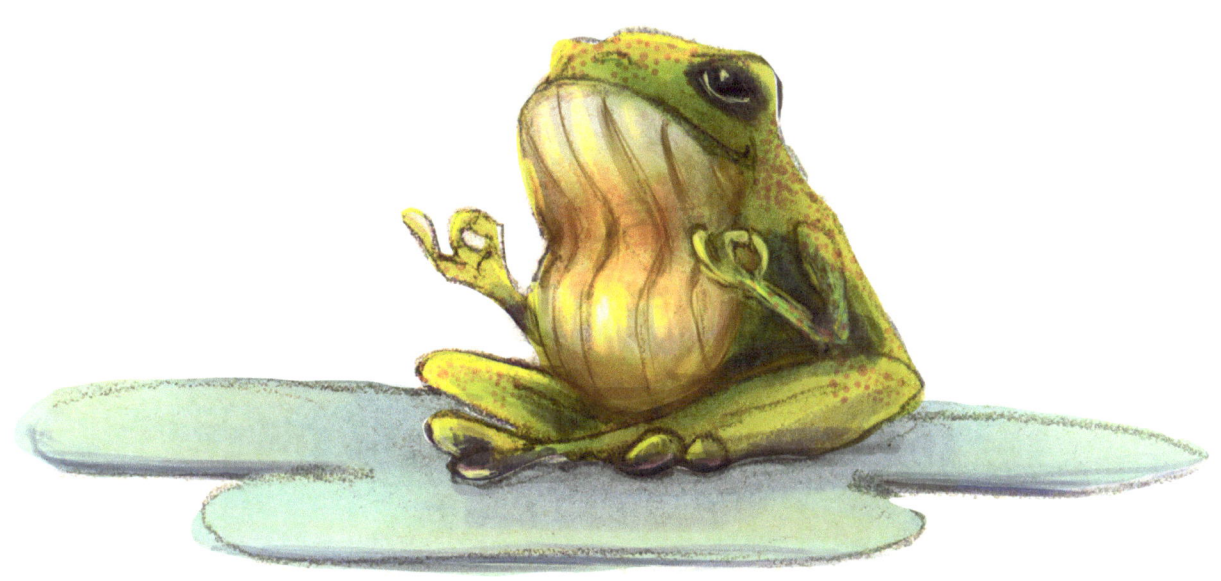

"The only mistake you can make in meditation? Not starting."

And as a parent, if you can find just a few moments to still your body and find peace in your mind, you are rewarded in multiples because these seconds of serenity refuel your ability to operate from calm intuition, improving things for everyone around you. PLUS, when your children see you practicing any mindful skill, you are modeling for them to do the same.

If you achieve even a hint of calm presence in your daily life, you're doing it right. There are no mistakes as you attempt to learn mindfulness. And the very act of seeking it counts!

Go to kindfulkids.com for ideas on creating KindfulKids Moments that can have big impact over time.

51

KindfulKids Fun Sheet

Draw pictures or use words to fill in the questions below

I am:

My favorite KindfulKids character is:

My favorite yoga pose is:

My favorite way to relax and be calm is:

The way I feel after this book is:

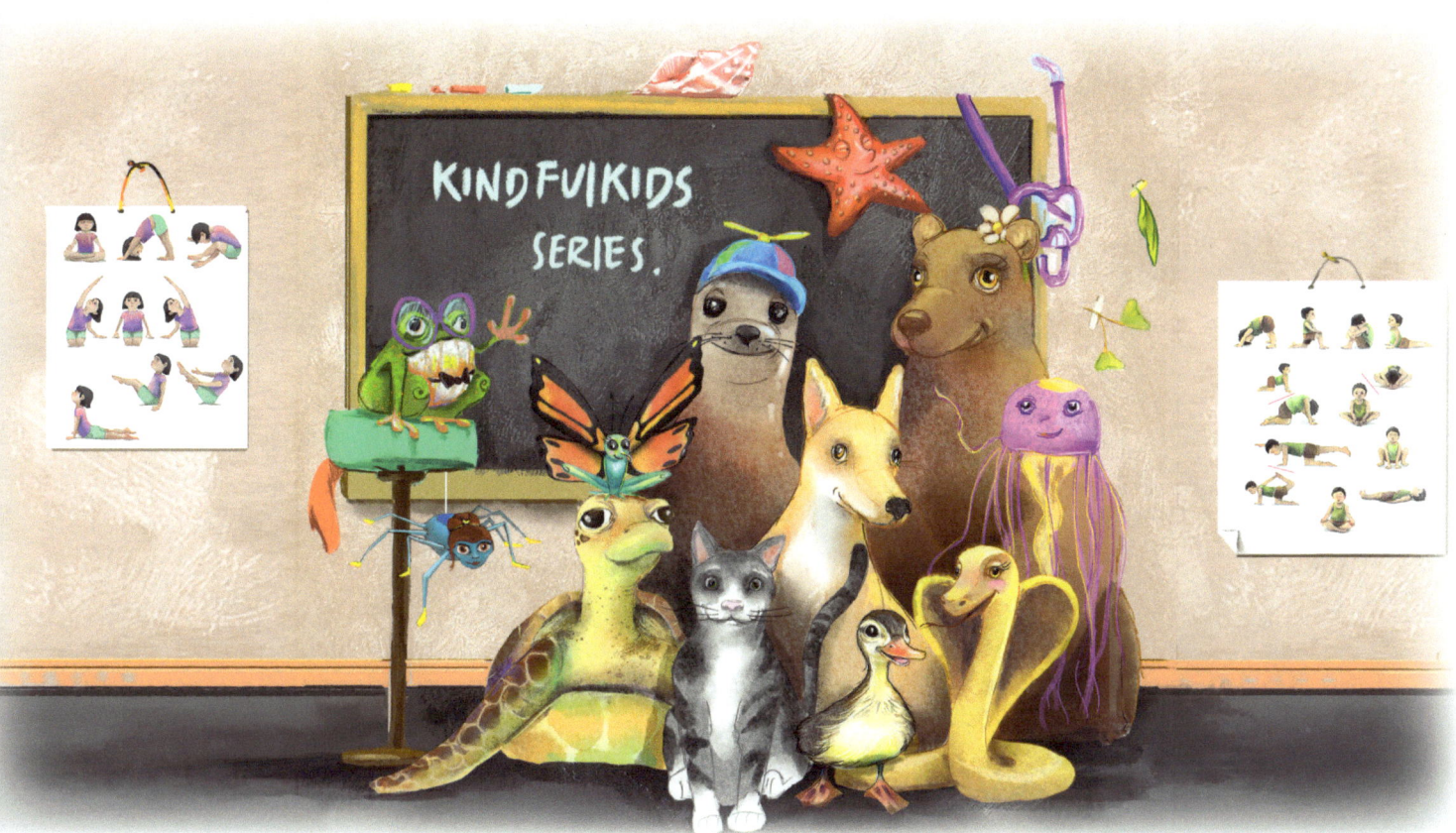

Thank you for being part of raising a generation of KindfulKids.

To learn more about the KindfulKids characters and receive
a free gift, "Kindful Moments With Our Kids"
visit kindfulkids.com

For any questions, comments or if you would like to order books
in quantity, please e-mail patricia@kindfulkids.com.

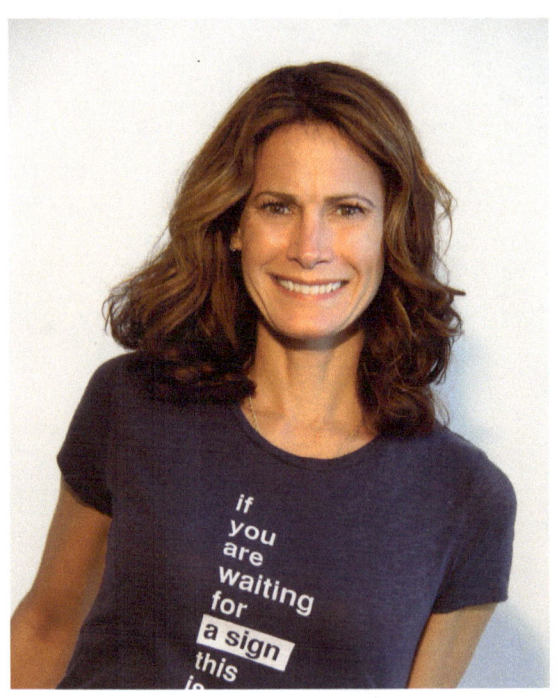

Patricia Leitch is an author and teacher who believes early introduction to relaxation and mindfulness practices are critical for kids to succeed in today's media-fueled world. During her teaching years in the California public school system, Patricia realized young kids grasped yoga poses and mindful techniques best when they were taught by adorable and funny animal characters. Thus, the creation of Danny the Dingo Dog, Freddy the Wise Frog, and their adventures around Pondering Pond.

This book is part of the KindfulKids Adventure Series that aims to engage children with steady and meaningful lessons to build an authentic mindfulness practice. Children enjoy the stories featuring cool creatures, practicing yoga poses and learning breathing and meditation techniques. The books explore kindness, emotional regulation, calming and focus techniques, gratitude, growth mindset, and other social emotional topics that support academic and life success. For more information, go to kindfulkids.com.

Soledad Cook is a scientist and an illustrator who understands the importance of delivering complex messages through illustrations. She loves the art of storytelling and her illustrations are full of life. They are made with the sole purpose of taking the young reader to another world where they can meet characters and learn new things.

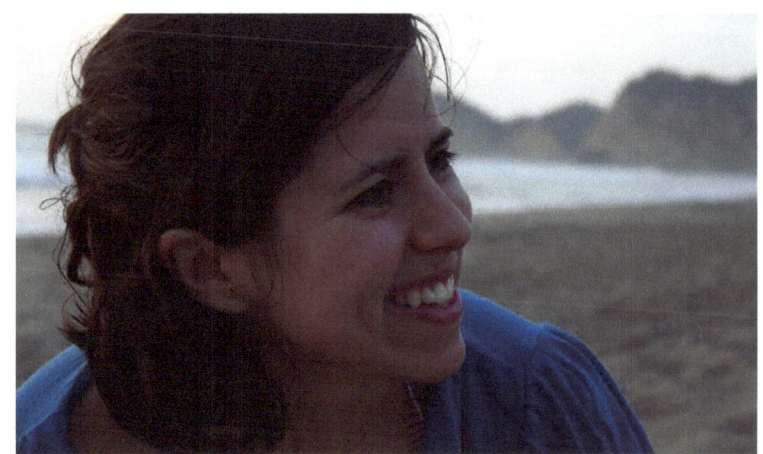